Shattered

Shattered

Life with ME

Lynn Michell

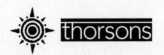

Thorsons
An Imprint of HarperCollins*Publishers*
77–85 Fulham Palace Road
Hammersmith, London W6 8JB

The website address is:
www.thorsonselement.com

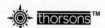

and *Thorsons* are trademarks of
HarperCollins*Publishers* Ltd

First published 2003

10 9 8 7 6 5 4 3 2 1

A catalogue record of this book
is available from the British Library

ISBN 0 00 715503 4

Printed and bound in Great Britain by
Creative Print and Design (Wales), Ebbw Vale

For the memory of my mother

Contents

Acknowledgements

This book is narrated by many voices. In the hope that others would benefit from their experiences, men, women and young people opened their hearts and talked through pain and exhaustion to give me an insight into lives changed and diminished by ME. As I wrote, they were by my side. During times when my own health was low, and the project was left untouched, recollections of those fine people urged me back to the manuscript to pick up the threads. None of you are named here. You know who you are. I thank you all from the bottom of my heart.

Dr Vance Spence, you have inspired me with your unfaltering belief that one day ME will be understood. Thank you for your readiness to leap in and help, for your faith in this project, and your e-mail avalanches of purple Irish prose.

This manuscript started life at about a million words. Dr Neil Abbot, Research Director of MERGE, chopped it up and edited it with skill and sensitivity until it resembled a book. Thank you, Neil, for making me smile every morning with your silly e-mail jokes as we worked on the book together.

Thank you Bente-Helène van Lambalgan, brave ME warrior and writer, for reading my manuscript in a second language and finding the flaws. Thank you for your loving friendship, for finding the yellow scarf in Amsterdam, and for all those e-hugs.

Thank you Theodora Bayly, Ciara MacLaverty, Cherry Headley, Dorothy Entwistle, Gillian Palmer, Cindy Cunningham and Helen Boden. Each of you understands ME; each of you has helped me in a unique way.

To my sister Patty – sorry for the years of tearful phone calls; thank you for your uncomplaining support, your emotional strength, the Oxfam parcels of clothes, and the new knickers when I was too ill to get to the shops.

Finally, my family: A thousand thanks and apologies to my son Nye – you resolved my stupidities on the computer, helped code the 300 pages of manuscript, and listened with patience and insight to endless extracts. Your wisdom, stoicism and love mean so much. Thank you Keith. Over sixteen years, your broad shoulders have taken on the burden of caring for three family members with ME. To readers who are also carers, need I say more? You have remained yourself – wise, calm, and funny. And Jo. Thank you for giving us hope because after three years you got better. It is a joy to know you live an ordinary and extraordinary life after ME.

I am grateful to Dr Charles Shepherd and the ME Association Small Grants Committee for providing funding for the research which formed the basis of this book.

Foreword

I can think of no other illness where such a powerful schism exists between those who suffer from it and those whose responsibility is to care for them. How can it be that an illness that affects between 100,000 and 200,000 persons of all ages in the United Kingdom and maybe as many as one million people in the United States of America is no longer referred to in medical textbooks, is not cited in medical research indexing systems and rarely features in the syllabus of undergraduate education in medical schools? Why have the experiences of these patients been largely ignored, their testimonies undervalued, even ridiculed, and their requests for assistance met often with prejudice and disbelief? An answer to this conundrum can be found in this scholarly account of the ME enigma.

Dr Lynn Michell has written a remarkable book – the product of her own experience as both an ME sufferer and a medical sociologist. For the first time, the authentic voices of people with ME are heard. Lynn Michell threads their narratives together expertly into a rich tapestry that highlights the central themes which dominate this illness: the lack of a recognised diagnosis; the scepticism of medical professionals; the lack of support from family and friends; the deserts of fatigue and pain; the loneliness involved in the search for help and empathy. These are not the voices of professionals with careers to promote; rather they are the voices of real people with terrible stories to tell. While people with ME and their carers will read this book and empathise, it should also be read by health and social care professionals for the insights that it gives.

Only scientific research into the causes and treatment of ME can prevent experiences like those described in this book. That comparatively little biomedical research has been done is due, in part, to the economics of medical research funding. In addition, ME has been subsumed by the all-inclusive diagnostic construct termed chronic fatigue syndrome (CFS). For most ME patients, the CFS term is insulting – akin to tuberculosis being renamed chronic cough syndrome – as it focuses on one symptom, 'fatigue', which is the hallmark of a range of illnesses with different underlying physiological causes. Nevertheless, the construction of the CFS label has resulted in a disproportionate allocation of funding towards psychosocial models of the illness. It has been left to a small minority of pioneer researchers – funded by smaller charities such as MERGE – to identify the physiological causes of ME and try to find a cure. Thanks to their efforts, some intriguing new developments are taking place in a variety of research centres throughout the world.

Lynn Michell's book reminds us that until specific treatments are found, real people will be affected by ME, often in catastrophic ways. Yet, the tales are not simply about broken lives – they also tell of survival and hope in the face of terrible adversity. Although people with ME may be *Shattered*, the stories in this book offer them the strength and courage to rebuild their lives.

DR VANCE A SPENCE

CHAIRMAN

MERGE (ME RESEARCH GROUP FOR EDUCATION AND SUPPORT)

Preface

It is March 1987. I am living in Edinburgh and working in Fife as an educational psychologist. It is an ordinary, happy – if somewhat hectic – life with two working parents and two young sons. There is a flu bug doing the rounds which floors me, my sons (then aged 6 and 12) and three members of my husband's academic department. But instead of slowly pulling out of our ill and exhausted states, none of us get better. The other adults take between one and ten years to regain their health. It will take three years for my elder son to recover. My younger son and I are still ill sixteen years later.

As weeks and then months passed, each of us realised that this was no ordinary viral infection which would run its self-limiting course but something different, difficult and extraordinarily debilitating. Nothing in my past experience of illness helped me understand what was happening to me. We already knew a couple of people who were ill with something called ME. It was not long before we suspected that we probably had the same thing. However, knowing a little about ME, even knowing someone with ME, did not prepare us for what was in store. Without the others for support, and in the face of rudeness, ignorance and hostility from the medical and teaching professions, I do not know how I would have pulled through those first years. But it took much longer for me to understand the nature of the illness, and longer still to work out how to manage and finally to get on top of it.

The road to recovery was different for each of us – just as it is for the people who tell their stories in these pages. My elder son needed a year off school, returned half-time for a further year, then recovered relatively quickly. My younger son remained ill throughout his schooling. He missed two complete years at primary school and attended half-time during the other years. With the move to secondary school came a steady deterioration in his health until, during standard grade exams, he suffered a profound relapse which left him bedbound. He is still clawing his way out, but now, seven years on, he is finally making progress.

It took me three years to become half-human, and seven years altogether to regain 75 per cent of my previous health and energy – at which point I made a disastrously wrong decision. I took on a full-time research fellowship in a MRC (Medical Research Council) unit in Glasgow. The work was rewarding; the workplace seductive and stimulating after years of solitude. The first year went well, although I spent most evenings and weekends resting. But early into the second year, with the added strain of family problems, symptoms returned and I ignored them. At the end of the second year I went under. The relapse was severe compared with the start of the illness. For a year I was bedbound and paralysed down my right arm. I was a write-off – physically, mentally and emotionally. It has taken me another seven years altogether to climb part-way out of the pit and this time my recovery has been much slower.

This account of my own illness explains the 'I' who tells this story. There is a paradox about being both inside and outside the narrative but it seems the best way to do it. Because I share with the other people who tell their stories an illness with a monumental impact on life quality, it felt wrong to leave out my own voice. I understand ME too. I decided to draw on that shared experience and empathy, rather than ignore it. So I too am present in the text, throwing in bits of my own story and adding my own comments where they serve to clarify and add to the experiences of others. I have tried to be present, but not intrusive.

I could have written an autobiographical account of my illness, but one of the less obvious aspects of ME is the way it deals out a slightly different hand of cards each time it strikes. Of course, there are common elements in the pattern of symptoms and in people's interactions with the non-sick world, but in other ways no two sufferers are exactly alike. A single story of the illness would offer only part of the picture. I needed many voices to do justice to the complexity of ME and to describe the diverse ways in which lives are lessened and altered. Instead of a single narrative thread, there is a weaving together of many stories.

This book is for everyone who has ME. It is for those who have had ME in the past. It is for carers and others involved in the lives of sufferers. In these pages, people with ME will recognise others who suffer and live and feel and react just as they do. They will find acknowledgement and validation. I hope that they will find support in the knowledge that they are far from alone.

I hope too that this book will have a wider appeal and interest for clinicians and academics who ponder issues concerning the social acceptability of illness and the way a disease's status and meaning can change over time and with medical understanding and knowledge. In this sense, I am writing not just about an illness called ME but about the human condition.

Introduction

*Still we hope that some improvement will hit us like a
ship out of the fog.*
CIARA MACLAVERTY

ME is different from cancer or heart disease or diabetes.
They are at least partly understood and so are acceptable
and real. ME does not yet have a pigeonhole in the medical
sorting office. Because it is not understood it is not legiti-
mised. For this reason, I cannot write about ME without
writing about the social stigma attached to it. The mythology which began in the early days with taunts about 'yuppie
flu' still haunts people with ME. They have been pushed
underground and silenced, not only by the circumscription
of illness but by jeering criticism about the legitimacy of
their diagnosis and their suffering. This book is about an illness at a particular time and in a particular social context. In
a climate of medical shoulder-shrugging ME is linked to just
about everything from previous behaviours, inappropriate
attitudes, personality problems, to a 'need to be ill'. People
with ME are described as 'over-achievers', 'driven', 'over-
sensitive' and, most patronising, 'four-star people with five-
star ambitions'. What is written here puts the record straight.
People with ME are very ill and very heroic. They face a
medical profession and a society which reflect back to them

a skewed and inaccurate perception of their suffering. ME is a serious, organic illness, yet sometimes it seems that those who suffer from it are the only ones who know that.

Those with ME are keen to tell their stories, no matter how ill they are and how tired they become after talking for a long time. Their narratives spill out like burst dams because, for once, away from the doctor's surgery, the consultant's clinic or the guidance teacher's room, away from people who are cynical, bored or disbelieving, they are offered a sympathetic and supportive context in which to speak. The mismatch between how people really feel and how others think they feel, is one of the strongest themes in this book, as Chloe, one of the subjects, explains:

◆ I just wish doctors would be a bit more understanding, even if they don't believe in ME. They must realise their patient is unwell. This is what gets me. If they would just look at your life, and listen. I was very active; why on Earth would I want to be ill? I want my life back. I want to go to work. I want to be normal. Do you know what I mean? How can they think you're trying to skive? Why does no one listen? If there was just someone there to talk to, but people don't understand.

And so this is a human story rather than a medical one, or at least it is a medical story only in so far that it is about what happens when the medical profession does not yet understand a particular illness. It is about the way lives change when people become ill with a bewildering and demoralising illness which is not regarded as 'real'. It is about how it *feels* to be deeply, bizarrely ill. It is about fruitless dialogues with a disbelieving society; about the attitudes of the non-sick; about relationships, loss and self-identity; about the need for support; and different ways of managing and coming through the other side. It describes the impact of an illness which drastically alters everyday living, even alienating friends, relatives and colleagues. Writing about chronic illness, Wells[1] says that it comes without an instruction manual. ME comes without an agreed name; CFS, PVFS or, in the United States, CFIDS. It comes without a diagnostic test; without hope of a cure; or relief from a terrible rainbow of symptoms. But it comes with questions: Is this a single illness? Is it a real illness? Is it all in the mind? When and how will it end? It brings a legacy of lingering fear because relapses are frequent.

The people who tell their stories here are men, women and young people from Scotland and California. Their ages range from 14 to 67 years. They have had ME for between two and eighteen years. Some have recovered completely and so reflect on their experiences. Some hang on, at great personal cost, to a semblance of normal life. Some have retreated to the ME ghetto, avoiding the healthy because to interact with them is too difficult. Some are housebound and severely disabled. They include a firefighter, a GP, a university professor, a librarian, a dairy worker, a car mechanic, an artist, a storyteller, two musicians, a therapist, an audio-typist and a number of very articulate students. Their collective and individual voices disabuse us of ME as 'yuppie flu' or 'all in the mind', and banish the stereotype of the middle-aged, neurotic female which is perpetuated by the collusion of ignorant doctors and a careless media.

Telling it how it is

The transcripts show that ME is more than a list of symptoms; it brings social and personal change on a scale unimaginable to the healthy. What stands out for me, reading the transcripts and remembering the interviews, is the totality and comprehensiveness of the disruption and devastation of day-to-day lives, such as Phil's:

> I've lost my pride, self-respect and confidence, that's top of the list ... I can't look forward to settling down with that special person, having a family. I feel that opportunity is being lost to me with every year that passes and that saddens me a lot ... I've lost finance, all my life savings have gone, I'm living on 70 quid a week, abject poverty. Some days I don't eat. Some days I go without heat. You know, it's that basic.

In previous studies, researchers have defined life quality in a variety of ways, measuring levels of physical activity or social activity, employment or housing, loss of income, loss of self-esteem and sexual satisfaction.[2] When the interviewees talk about the destruction of life quality, they mean all of these and much more. They talk about the loss of physical, social and emotional well-being; about the erosion of self-worth; about the loss of a sense of self. This is how ME changes life quality, not in one or two ways, but totally, deeply, comprehensively.

There are common themes and issues which emerge again and again, such as isolation, ways of coping, loss and an uncertain future. But for each person, ME also has its own particular meaning. For several, it is the loss of physical stamina and fitness. For another, the faltering of a fine intellect. For another, coming to terms with childlessness. Or the reining in of a creative, exuberant personality and the acceptance of emotional blandness. For a few people, however – mainly women – ME means the opportunity to take stock, change direction, and embrace a different life.

A stigmatised illness

So far there is no definitive diagnostic test for ME. There is no litmus test which will tell a doctor whether an individual has ME or not, although trials now reveal a number of physical differences between groups of people who have ME and control groups who do not. Without a test, ME is still regarded by many doctors as not 'real' and, by default, 'all in the mind'. The rare doctor who does believe in it may be branded and ridiculed by his colleagues, as Alistair, the GP in this study, explains:

◆ It's a no-win situation really. You've got this condition that can be totally disabling and yet it is not accepted. A lot of my colleagues don't want to get involved with it. You get bogged down in a lot of paperwork and verbiage, and they're often having to put down a diagnosis which they don't believe in. Sometimes you get branded as a bit of an open-toed sandled, faded jeans type because you may believe in ME. We'd feel a lot better with a test because then we could say, 'Look we've got a diagnosis. We haven't got this uncertainty.' I think we'd all love it.

For the interviewees, living with such misunderstanding and scepticism hurts almost as much as their symptoms, and this explains why they keep searching for something – or somebody – to validate their experience.

ME patients now are where sufferers of multiple sclerosis, TB and rheumatoid arthritis were before the physiological bases of their illnesses were identified. These illnesses were once misunderstood as psychological disorders and personality weaknesses when they were at the same stage in their medical evolution. Susan Sontag, writing about TB, describes how the illness was shrouded with myths and metaphors: 'TB was understood, like insanity, to be a one-sidedness: a failure of will or an over-intensity'.[3] She quotes a textbook definition of TB, written before its cause was discovered, as 'hereditary disposition, unfavourable climate, sedentary lifestyle, defective ventilation, deficiency of light, and depressing emotions'.[4] This is where ME is now, relegated to the psychiatric slush pile, and it will remain there until a medical breakthrough re-writes history. And referring to the rising popularity of 'trash psychology' which gives every lay person the right to decide whether people with ME are truly ill or not, Munson writes, 'Nobody has partaken in such a zealous barrage of metaphoric lampoons since the nineteenth-century days of multiple sclerosis, which was called in its early days "hysterical paralysis".'[5]

The lack of a diagnostic test is largely responsible for the huge discrepancy between the experience of the illness and the inadequacy of the support and understanding offered by those who treat, observe and write about it. 'At the turn of the millennium, the public still lacks a real grasp on what CFIDS patients are dealing with. Because of illusions that CFIDS is simply a disease of tired people ... the public has been largely deprived of accurate information.'[6]

Dialogues with a disbelieving society

Most doctors don't like ME. Sceptical and unconvinced, they are often reluctant to offer a diagnosis confirming ME, as Alistair explains:

◆ I could easily have been one of those sceptics. When I got ME it was in the age of yuppie flu so we were all trained to be a bit sceptical. People will turn up feeling hellish and just be told, 'Don't be silly,' or 'Here's your antidepressant, it's a depressive illness you've got.'

What doctors and other professionals do not grasp is the enormous impact of their behaviour on the patients; it is within their power either to help people find a way through their ordeal, or to make an already tough illness doubly difficult. A supportive GP can make all the difference in the world. The current medical view of ME filters down into society's attitudes: if doctors say people with ME are malingerers, then most people, including relatives and friends, accept this to be the truth. In the wake of inaccurate accounts by doctors come emotive media reports, dismissive attitudes in schools and other institutions, and hurtful, inappropriate behaviour from family and friends. Young people, in particular, have a very hard time as they battle with indifference, disbelief, taunts and bullying. The narratives here show how misguided, negative views of ME profoundly affect the everyday lives of sufferers.

These narratives also reveal interesting gender differences in the search for validation. In general, women experience more hostility and disbelief than men, although the story is not simple or clear cut. Probably reflecting their status in society, young people have the hardest time of all. They are subjected to the worst advice, the least appropriate treatments and the harshest criticism.

Relationships

As with any serious, chronic illness, ME upsets the domestic apple cart. It places an enormous burden on everyone in the family, causing tension and heartache as a once fit and fully-contributing member of the family becomes a lifeless figure on the sofa for months and years on end. Everything changes. There is no forward-planning, no holidays to look forward to, no outings, no normal family life. Wives, husbands and children try to carry on as usual, but there is no avoiding the visible truth of a loved one who has had to withdraw from family life.

In general, the men who are sick have an easier time in the domestic arena than the women. Men are more likely to be left in peace to get better as their women folk look after them in every possible way, taking over childcare and domestic duties. In contrast, most ill women continue to orchestrate the running of the household from their beds. Young people battle with the conflicting emotions of gratitude to their parents for taking care of them when they have to return home, and guilt for not wanting to be in that situation.

Having someone who truly understands and sympathises can make a world of difference. Relatives and friends can offer lifelines or they can turn their backs. And, as many people discovered, being ill quickly sorts out those who truly care. Many people report that only a few loyal friends and relatives stick by them. Being ill is a lonely business. Caring for a loved one with ME is a lonely business. But that loneliness is intensified when relatives and friends keep up the pretence that nothing much is wrong and nothing much has changed.

Relationships can wither and die as ME takes a stronger and stronger hold. Josh, an 18-year-old student, has been housebound for three years. In that time he has been too ill to interact with people who expect him to behave 'normally', and so all contact with his peer group has ceased. Too ill to meet friends or talk on the phone, he has lived the life of a hermit. He has endured complete social isolation, as well as pain, fatigue, insomnia, brain fog, nausea, and the myriad other physical and cognitive symptoms that are familiar to everyone who is severely affected. One of the most important reasons for writing this book is to highlight the plight of Josh, the other six young people, and the thousands of uncounted, unheard children and adolescents who wait alone at a red light which does not change.

Coping strategies

To write about the impact of an illness is one side of the coin. The other is to describe how individuals respond to, and cope with, fundamental and long-term change. The people here say that they are navigating uncharted waters. Nothing in their previous experience of illness prepared them for it. To understand their responses, we have to appreciate that they are operating with a different mindset. ME is not like acute illnesses, nor many chronic ones for which there is a test, a diagnosis and treatment. Patients with other illnesses may be just as ill, but they can usually be given some statistically based information about prognosis, recovery and expected life quality. But people with ME face an open-ended and uncertain future. For instance, a nurse who became ill in one of the earliest outbreaks at the Royal Free Hospital in London is as ill today, fifty years on, as she was then.[7] As just one case history, she may be unrepresentative of the population with ME, but we have no way of knowing how unrepresentative.

The people here talk about the way they deal with the shock and how they respond in the early stages, banging their heads against unyielding walls, and running from therapy to therapy as they search for understanding, diagnosis, treatment, cure and support. Later, as the grim reality of the illness settles in, they adapt to its demands by trying out ways of coping. Different strategies work for different people, but they all have their roots in the lack of a diagnostic test, and the lack of a validation of experience. In this context, every response is understandable, even if some are unproductive. Responses to ME range from denial, to a search for treatment, to adaptation, to positive gain. Some people are just well enough to cling on to what is central in their lives, like Fraser, who somehow kept working as a fire-fighter:

◆ No, I didn't look for anyone to lean on. I wanted to be treated just the same because I was trying to keep my work as one bit of my life that was still ticking over. I'd lost my rugby. I wasn't going to lose my work. There was no point in the health nurse coming to talk to me for half an hour because she couldn't do a bloody thing about it anyway – so I just tried to keep soldiering on.

Others, because they are so ill, such as Alison and her partner, redefine the meaning of 'normal' and retreat to the ME ghetto away from the world of the well:

◆ The great benefit of being a couple with it is that we're never comparing ourselves with normal people. We're normal. The rest of the world isn't.

Individuals may run the gamut of these responses before coming to terms with long-term disability. Then, often, comes acceptance, clawing back, clever management and, finally, some degree of control over fluctuating symptoms and energy levels. Intuitively, they work at maintaining the delicate balance between doing too much and not doing enough, juggling rest and activity, until they can maintain an equilibrium of health. People with ME become skilled harvesters of energy, accepting that they may never reach previous levels of physical and emotional stamina but nevertheless finding satisfaction in their lives. Less becomes more. For most people, ME means a different way of living.

These five themes which emerge from the interviews, discussions and self-help group meetings form the framework of this book. Together they give a representative picture of what it is like to have ME, of what it is like to have one's symptoms regarded as trivial or unreal. For all that, through the distress and tragedy of the accounts, we find incredible courage, resourcefulness, resilience and humour.

Because I am ill myself, it has taken a long time to write this book. During the four years of its preparation, there are signs that attitudes to ME are starting to change. With the recent publication of the Chief Medical Officer's Report has come a first public statement that ME is a serious illness. While this, and future research, will be slow to have an impact on society's attitudes and behaviours – as the history of other 'mystery' illnesses prove – perhaps those with ME can now dare to hope for more tolerance and understanding instead of heartbreaking hostility.

The people with ME

The profiles outlined here describe the participants at the time of interview. An up-date of their progress is given in the final part of the book, 'Postscript: Facing the Future – Four Years On' (see p. 279).

In Edinburgh and a Midlothian rural village

THE WOMEN
Denise

Age 48. Onset was sudden after a viral infection in 1997. At worst 80 per cent disabled; now 60 per cent. Diagnosed by an alternative practitioner. Denise used to work full-time as a secretary, but is currently unable to work except for an hour a day on playground duty at the local school. She receives Income Support but cannot face the hassle and exhaustion involved in applying for Incapacity Benefit.

Chloe

Age 32. Onset was sudden after two consecutive viral infections in 1994. At worst 80 per cent disabled; now 60 per cent. Her sister who is a nurse suggested ME, a diagnosis which was later confirmed by a private medical consultant. Chloe used to work full-time as a typist but is now unable to work at all. She receives Incapacity Benefit but has been refused Disability Living Allowance and feels she hasn't the strength to go through the appeals procedure.

May

Age 50. Onset was gradual during 1990 with no precipitating factors except, possibly, long-term stress. Was ill for two years. At worst 75 per cent disabled; now fully recovered. A GP confirmed her self-diagnosis of ME. May was unable to work for a year, but is now back doing the accounts and helping with the family dairy delivery business. May's husband was also diagnosed as having ME. May did not apply for benefits.

Lizzie

Age 33. Onset was sudden after an acute viral illness in 1985. Was ill for four years. At worst 80 per cent disabled; now almost fully recovered, but she still has to take care. Self-diagnosis confirmed by a private practitioner after reading information and literature about ME. Liz is working full time as a therapist. She did not apply for benefits.

Janet

Age 67. Onset was sudden after a series of viral infections in 1982. Is still ill after seventeen years. At worst 90 per cent dis-abled; now 40 per cent. Self-diagnosis later confirmed by private practitioner. Janet is a doctor's wife who was a full-time homemaker and mother of four young children when she became ill. Her children are now grown up. She is not eligible for benefits.

Fiona
Age 45. Onset was sudden after a viral illness in 1985. Was ill for two years. At worst 60 per cent disabled; now 5 per cent. Diagnosed by NHS consultant. Fiona has returned to work full-time as an administration officer. She did not apply for benefits because she was able to return to work after sick leave.

Alison
Age 48. Onset was sudden after using head lice pesticide shampoo containing lindane in 1992. Is still ill after eight years. At worst 90 per cent disabled; now 60 per cent. Diagnosed by GP. Alison used to work as a musician and teacher, but has been unable to work since 1992. A year after she became ill, her partner, also a musician, developed ME symptoms and has been unable to work for the past seven years. Alison receives Incapacity Benefit and Disability Living Allowance, although she has been through several appeals and tribunals during her eight years of illness.

THE MEN
Mike
Age 41. Onset was sudden after a viral infection in 1992. Was ill for eighteen months. At worst 60 per cent disabled; now 10 per cent (unable to do heavy physical work or strenuous

exercise, and still alcohol intolerant). Diagnosed by GP. Managed to keep working as a surveyor by doing less, by resting and working flexible hours. He is now working full-time again.

Liam
Age 62. Onset was sudden after a viral illness in 1984. Was seriously ill for a year, followed by gradual, partial recovery. At worst 60 per cent disabled; now fluctuates between 5 per cent and 15 per cent. Diagnosed by GP and confirmed by NHS hospital consultant. Managed to keep working as a university professor, although during the worst months he took time off, reduced his hours and worked only on essential teaching and research projects. He is now working full-time but feels he is not fully recovered.

Fraser
Age 40. Onset was sudden after a chest infection in 1989. Was ill for between four and five years. At worst 40 per cent disabled; now fully recovered. Diagnosed by GP. Managed to keep working as a firefighter by doing nothing else. While ill, was unable to continue former training as a rugby player or to take part in any physical exercise.

Phil
Age 40. Onset sudden after a viral illness and stress in 1987. Is still ill after twelve years. At worst 90 per cent disabled; now 50 per cent. Self-diagnosis later confirmed by GP. Phil was working long hours as a youth worker when he became ill. He has been unable to work since 1987, although he

works part-time at home for ME support groups, and has completed various part-time courses. He receives Incapacity Benefit and Disability Living Allowance, although he has had to cope with a number of refusals and appeals.

Jamie
Age 56. Onset gradual following a viral infection and stress from 1989 onwards. Is still ill after ten years. At worst 80 per cent disabled; now 25 per cent. He diagnosed himself; later reluctantly confirmed by GP. Jamie used to work as a teacher, children's writer and illustrator, artist, historian and storyteller. He has published several books. He has been unable to work since 1989, although, when able, he is active in the local history society, and reads and tells stories to groups of children in one-off events. He receives Incapacity Benefit.

Alistair
Age 56. Onset sudden with no precipitating factors. Was ill for six years. At worst 40 per cent disabled; now fully recovered. As a GP, he recognised his illness as ME, and had his diagnosis confirmed by a hospital consultant. Alistair managed to keep working as a GP throughout his illness, although at his worst he was only just managing.

Ray
Age 27. Onset gradual from 1997 after prolonged stress at work. Is still ill after two years and is possibly deteriorating. At worst 40 per cent disabled; now 40 per cent. Diagnosed by NHS hospital consultant. Ray used to work as a sports car mechanic and raced at weekends. He was setting up his

own business when he became ill. He has been unable to work at all since 1997. He receives Incapacity Benefit and Income Support.

THE YOUNG PEOPLE

I had to make a decision about where the cut-off point was between adults and young people. Children in their early teens were clearly children, but what about the young people in their twenties? Were they adults or young people? In the end, I used the age of the person at the onset of illness as my criterion. An individual was classified as a young person if they became ill while they were still studying, either at school or in higher education, and their education remained disrupted or non-existent, even if the individual was much older by the time they were interviewed. All the young people were stalled both in terms of their education and their social development. The youngest, Ruby, is 14. The oldest, Chris, is 30, but became ill ten years earlier while working as an agricultural student. One of the sickest, he has been housebound ever since, and so in his own words, feels 'stuck at 20'. While chronologically ten years older now, in terms of the experiences he has missed compared with his peers, he has hardly moved on. The other five students are aged between 18 and 22.

Rachel
Age 18. Sudden onset in 1991, struggled on part-time at school for several years before a total collapse in 1994. Is still ill after eight years. At worst 99.9 per cent disabled; now 80 per cent. Eventually diagnosed by a psychiatrist as having

CFS, but not ME. Mostly housebound, and cared for by her parents, she needs a wheelchair to get around and is often confined to bed. Rachel has been too ill for any kind of education for the past five years. Receives Incapacity Benefit and the mobility and care components of Disability Living Allowance, although she has been refused Disability Living Allowance several times.

Josh

Age 18. Gradual onset from the age of 6. Struggled on, attending less than half-time for his entire school career, and missing several complete years before a total collapse in 1998. Is still ill after thirteen years. At worst 99 per cent disabled; now 85 per cent. Eventually diagnosed by an NHS paediatric consultant at the age of 12. Since his relapse three years ago, Josh has been housebound, cared for by his parents, and is too ill for any form of education. Receives Severe Disability Allowance and Disability Living Allowance.

Kirsty

Age 22. Sudden onset after a viral illness in 1991. Struggled on at school until 1993 when she was studying for six Highers, when, after a marked deterioration in her health, she became too ill to continue her education. Is still ill after eight years. At worst 100 per cent disabled; now 50 per cent. Diagnosed in 1995 by Jan de Vries, an alternative practitioner in Scotland. Kirsty lives at home where she is supported and cared for by her parents. She is too ill to move into her own flat. She helps her sisters with childminding, but is otherwise unable to study or work. She receives Income Support.

Ruby

Age 14. Sudden onset after flu in 1996. Initially tried to manage part-time schooling but became too ill. Is still ill after two and a half years. At worst 100 per cent disabled; now 30 per cent. Has only recently received a diagnosis of ME from a private GP. Ruby also suffers from Attention Deficit Disorder which made for an interesting, brief and forthright interview. Ruby's mother, a single parent, was diagnosed as having Munchausen's syndrome by proxy, a rare condition in which a parent fabricates her child's symptoms to receive attention, and as a result has faced many bitter battles with the medical and educational establishments. Ruby is slowly recovering and now attends school part-time. Ruby's mother is too exhausted to apply for benefits.

Chris

Age 33. Sudden onset in 1989 after a viral infection which was perhaps triggered by eating his sandwich lunch in the pig pens while working as an agricultural student. Is still ill after ten years. At worst 75 per cent disabled; now 60 per cent. Eventually diagnosed by an ME specialist, eight years after becoming ill. His condition is described as 'atypical ME'. Chris is mostly housebound, although he manages to live in a shared flat and look after himself. He receives Income Support.

Jessie

Age 19. Sudden onset in 1992 after a viral infection. Is still ill after seven years, but is recovering. At worst 80 per cent disabled; now fluctuates between 30 per cent and 60 per cent. Diagnosed herself as having ME, a diagnosis later confirmed by an NHS hospital consultant. Jessie was still at school when she became ill but struggled on, working from home, and achieved excellent exam results. She made it to university, completed a year, then crashed and had to return home to be cared for by her parents. Recently she returned to university and has resumed her studies.

David
Age 22. Onset probably at age 7, after a severe chest infection, although ME symptoms remained mild for many years. He missed a complete year of education, then returned to school, never really well, until he was 14 when he suffered a total collapse after a viral infection. Is still ill after fifteen years. Has been too ill to receive any education since he was 14. At worst 100 per cent disabled; now 60 per cent. Diagnosed six months after his relapse by a hospital consultant as having Post Viral Fatigue Syndrome, not ME. David lives at home and is cared for by his mother, now a single parent after her husband moved out of the family home. David was too ill to be interviewed. His story is told by his mother Marilyn.

IN CALIFORNIA
Chrissie
Age 42. Onset sudden after a viral illness. Has been ill for ten years. At worst 80 per cent disabled; recovered to a level where she could function well, but is now 80 per cent disabled again after a severe relapse. Diagnosed by her physician. Formally a secretary and artist but now unable to work at all, Chrissie lives in fear of losing her home and is fighting an ongoing battle with her health insurance company.

Dawn

Age 45. Onset sudden after a viral illness. Ill for fourteen years. At worst 90 per cent disabled; now 40 per cent. Self-diagnosed. Dawn continued to work part-time as a paramedic, just managing by excluding nearly everything else in her life. Five years ago she suffered a severe stroke which left her unable to speak or walk. Brain damage has left her with language and mobility problems.

Ruth

Age 42. Onset sudden after a viral illness. Ill for eighteen years. At worst 100 per cent disabled. Recovered enough to return to work full-time as a librarian, but a sudden and dramatic relapse left her 100 per cent disabled again. Diagnosed by her physician as having fibromyalgia. Ruth is 80 per cent disabled and in constant severe pain, three years after her relapse. She lives in a spiritual community.

PARENTS AND CARERS

Marilyn
David's mother

Emily
Liam's wife

Ann
Ruby's mother

Nelson
Josh's father

OTHER CONTRIBUTORS

Dr Bruce Campbell

Sudden onset in 1997 after a viral infection. Ill for two and a half years. At worst 75 per cent disabled; now largely recovered. His self-diagnosis was quickly confirmed by his personal physician. He had been a consultant to projects at the Stanford Medical School, including work with David Spiegel's group support research, the Arthritis Self-Help course and the Chronic Disease Self-Management course. He quickly concluded that conventional medicine had little to offer him, so set himself the task of developing self-help management techniques which would help him recover. He stresses the interaction of his own path to recovery and the development of the self-help groups which began in California and are now run on the Internet.

Ciara MacLaverty

Ciara MacLaverty was a student at Glasgow University when she became ill with sudden onset ME in 1986, aged 18. Severely affected for the rest of the 1980s she could do little more than exist. The early 1990s saw a partial remission that allowed her to study part-time and gain an Arts and Social Sciences degree. She tried creative writing and has had several short stories published in anthologies together with articles in newspapers.

After a relapse in the late 1990s she remains mostly bedbound, where she uses a laptop computer to help campaign for ME awareness. She enjoys reading, writing and seeing good friends when symptoms allow. Despite being continually challenged by the severity of her limitations, she hopes never to become an 'illness bore'.

PART 1

Telling it how it is

CHAPTER 1

What is ME?

It's stupid to call it Chronic Fatigue Syndrome. It should be called the Forever Dead Syndrome.
KEITH JARRETT. Jazz/classical pianist. Ill with ME for four years.

The most important contribution this book can make is to portray what ME is like from the inside. At least as relevant as all the discussions of causes, contributory factors and symptoms is an accurate account of what it is really like to live with the illness. This is where we should start. This is Phil talking about the experience of ME:

It would be difficult to imagine being any worse. I was at the stage of crawling on my hands and knees at times. I remember trying to answer the phone and not being able to get there quickly enough because I was crawling. I was confused by really simple things, and muddling my words and not being able to finish sentences. Just a complete mess cognitively. There was a great deal of weakness in my limbs, and a drained complexion and pallor. I was bedridden. I mean I was in bed 23 hours out of 24. I was sleeping at least 18 of those 23 hours. Extremely exhausted, extremely emotional, depressed certainly; partly a reaction to physiological illness, partly, I'm sure, due to alterations in my central nervous system. And yes, at times, suicidal.

ME broke upon the public consciousness a couple of decades ago as a mystery illness, an enigma or condition which was probably all in the mind. While some of this mythology lingers, a recent report by an independent working group to the Chief Medical Officer of England recognises it as a 'genuine illness [which] imposes a substantial burden on the health of the UK population. Improvement of health and social care for people affected by the condition is an urgent challenge.'[1] It affects women and men of all ages and from all walks of life and has a more comprehensive impact on life quality than almost any other chronic illness.[2] It can take years to reach even a partial level of recovery, yet we do not know what ME is, its cause or causes remain controversial, and treatment is elusive. It will take an imaginative leap and a rare kind of lateral thinking to piece together the puzzle that is ME.

This is not the place for a critique of medical hypotheses about the causes of ME, a detailed description of the enormous range of reported symptoms, or a list of the largely unsuccessful conventional and complementary treatments reported in clinical trials and anecdotal evidence. There are other books that do this job – and do it well – so only a brief account of the current state of play is included below. Instead, this book is about people's experiences of ME, a collective account of what it is like to live with the illness. This is the human story, not the medical one.

Current medical research

The state of research into ME is described by one reviewer as 'a fight':

> Fighting has broken out in one of the most volatile areas of medicine – chronic fatigue syndrome (CFS) or myalgic encephalopathy (ME). For more than a decade groups of disaffected patients have been challenging mainstream medical assumptions about the nature of this condition, which affects nearly 250,000 people in the UK. Now patients are furious because they believe that establishment psychiatrists have pulled off a pre-emptive grant strike that will make a mockery of government promises to give their objections a fair hearing. The fight also throws up important questions about who should decide priorities in research. [3]

While the controversy rages, several different hypotheses are emerging, though there is still a long way to go before we know what ME 'is' and how we can get better. In the search for an infectious cause, some scientists believe that we are dealing with an entirely new and powerful retrovirus; others believe that ME is related or linked to the family of enteroviruses and have commented on the likeness between ME and poliomyelitis. It may be that as a result of viral damage our immune systems no longer function normally so that symptoms usually associated with ongoing infection such as malaise, flu-like feelings, aches and pains, headaches and fever are frequently reported. It may be that the functioning of the central nervous system is fundamentally disrupted, producing cognitive impairment and sensory overload. Clinical tests show how the ability to retrieve, process, store and recover information is affected, thus offering some explanation as to why so many people with ME cannot do 'multi-tasking', and report difficulties with concentration and memory retrieval. Sensory input can be intolerable, with the ordinary world perceived as a nightmare arcade of glaring, flickering lights and shattering, nerve-fraying noise. Such symptoms are hard to describe and so often go unrecorded. Another line of investigation using sophisticated brain imaging suggests that the oxygen supply to the brain is reduced, producing symptoms that might be described as a slow, ongoing stroke.

All of this presents us with a complex picture with no clear hierarchy of cause and effect. Some symptoms may be the knock-on effect of damage further up the illness chain rather than the cause of the illness. Certainly, it is a far cry from the hopelessly inadequate description of ME as 'chronic fatigue'. Fatigue is associated with almost all chronic illnesses as well as with the aftermath of acute ones, but it describes only *one* of many symptoms. The distinction between fatigue and ME needs emphasising. If you are tired all the time, you do not have ME. If you are feeling drained following a viral illness but are recovering over weeks or months, you do not have ME. Post-viral fatigue is not the same as ME; nor is Chronic Fatigue Syndrome (which means only that people feel very tired for a long time for a variety of known and unknown reasons).

ME is not a good name, but it is the best we can do for now. Myalgic Encephalomyelitis means inflammation in the brain and spinal cord, even though there is little evidence that this is what is wrong with us. In the United States ME is called CFIDS (pronounced *Cee-Fids*) which stands for Chronic Fatigue Immune Dysfunction Syndrome. At a recent conference in Seattle,[4] doctors and patients agreed that that medics are now in a position to choose a new and more appropriate name which reflects what is known about the illness. Labels are important: they should be accurate and validating. Currently we have an inappropriate and inaccurate label but, because it is commonly used and recognised, I use it throughout the book to describe our condition.

Who gets ME?

As yet, no one has carried out a large-scale epidemiological study of ME using agreed diagnostic criteria – although such criteria do exist.[5] This is a real chicken-and-egg problem. How can scientists find out how many people are affected by this illness when there is no agreed definition of it? It is one thing counting people with green eyes or with a history of heart problems, but quite another counting people who are sick with a variably described and poorly understood disease in the absence of a definitive diagnostic test to separate those with ME from those with different fatiguing illnesses. However, using the available diagnostic criteria, one recent community-based study of 28,673 adults in the USA puts the proportion of the population affected at 0.42 per cent,[6] and a recent report by an independent working group to the Chief Medical Officer of England states that 'Overall, evidence suggests a population prevalence of at least

0.2 per cent–0.4 per cent'.[7] One American study carried out by the Centers for Disease Control in 1998 concluded that the incidence of ME is now higher than that for lung cancer, breast cancer or HIV infection in women.[8]

Men, women, young people and children of all ethnic groups and from all social backgrounds get ME. Various myths about ME take a long time to dispel – such as the one about ME affecting only white, affluent women – yet a study based in San Francisco found highest levels of the illness amongst African-Americans and Native Americans.[9] Another recent study in Chicago found that Latinos and those in the lower income groups are more, not less, likely to suffer from ME.[10]

Another belief is that women sufferers outnumber men by about 3 or 4:1, but a recent review of epidemiological studies concludes that there is only a 'slight' female–male predominance.[11] In the light of my own study this finding makes a lot of sense. The disparity may be a reporting phenomenon with men more reluctant to go to their GP or to acknowledge the severity of their condition. Or it may be that although roughly equal numbers of men and women become sick, the greater domestic support offered to men by their wives and partners means that they recover more quickly and do not plunge into the more severe and chronic forms of the illness. Either way – fewer men end up in consulting rooms to be counted.

Do all people with ME feel the same?

No two patients with ME are exactly alike. For some pain dominates; pain which feels as if it is grafted onto every bone and muscle in their bodies. For some there is weakness and exhaustion beyond anything most people can imagine. For others central nervous system disturbance is so disabling that the input from an environment such as a shop or a new room can produce sweating, dizziness, flu-like feelings and disorientation. Each of us seems to get a slightly different package, but the central, cardinal symptom for every person affected by ME is the tired-but-wired, heart-pounding malaise which returns after too much effort and exertion.

But don't ask what is too much, because often there is no easy or consistent answer. This is what we spend years of our lives trying to resolve. For a very ill person, too much can be taking a shower or making a sandwich. For someone further up the recovery ladder it may be a conversation too long, a walk too far or too prolonged a spell at the computer. For the nearly-well, it may be an inability to achieve a former level of physical fitness, or an awareness of reduced mental or emotional stamina. Yet despite our differences we usually recognise one another. It's not just the colour draining from our faces, or the botched sentences, or the need to lie down. It's what we say and the words we use to describe our condition. There is a common vocabulary and a shared experience which makes explanations unnecessary.

Onset

Having seen over 800 people with ME, Dr Charles Shepherd concludes that there are several kinds of onset.[12] Roughly 70 per cent of previously fit patients describe an acute onset which coincides with an infection but a failure to recover in the usual way. About 5 per cent of patients correlate the onset of ME with exposure to pesticides, chemical toxins or vaccinations; 10–15 per cent have no sudden onset and Shepherd concludes that these people, while fulfilling some of the internationally agreed criteria for ME such as fatigue, probably have some underlying psychiatric illness. Another 10 per cent either have an overlapping condition such as athletic overtraining syndrome, or are misdiagnosed and turn out to have a different diagnostic explanation for their chronic fatigue, such as a thyroid problem.

The distinction between sudden and gradual seems to be central in most discussions of onset. Either ME symptoms appear fairly rapidly and in some cases dramatically, or there is a more gradual and insidious onset with a general tiredness and malaise developing slowly into what is eventually labelled as ME. It is thought that most sudden onset cases follow a viral infection. Now some researchers believe that there may also be other triggers such as exposure to pesticides, or shock following a trauma such as a car accident. There seems to be some agreement that the prognosis for sudden onset ME is somewhat better than for gradual onset, but in the absence of an appropriate epidemiological study, we do not know how significant the difference is between these two beginnings. Up to now, the classification of ME into two types according to onset is only based on fairly small studies or on anecdotal evidence.

There are two points to be made here. First, there is the distinction between sudden and gradual onset. Some people go down with ME like a brick in the sea. There is no doubt, right from the start, that they are seriously ill in a way which is different from anything else they have experienced. Others gradually become ill over months or even years as ME takes hold. Second, there is the debate about whether ME is triggered by an infection – or indeed whether ME is itself an ongoing infection – or by other precipitating factors such as exposure to toxins and vaccinations. As yet there are no definite answers to any of these questions, but the majority of people, as Shepherd concludes, recall a triggering infection which coincided with the start of ME symptoms. This is how most people in my sample describe the onset of ME – an infection from which they do not recover. A minority of my interviewees describe their onset as gradual. Either they remember an infection or series of infections a long time in the past, then struggling on for a year or more, feeling awful, but they do not link the two events. Or they do not register a triggering infection at all, perhaps because there was none, perhaps because it was mild, perhaps because they were used to ignoring minor health problems. In my sample, two previously fit men fit this scenario. And in one case only, the gradual onset is described mainly in terms of depression and tiredness.

Of my sample, 10 of the 14 men and women remember the onset of ME as sudden. All but one also recall having an infection in the days or weeks prior to becoming ill. Liam, Chloe and Fiona had two bouts of flu from which they did not recover in the usual way. Phil had a series of infections.

Fraser had a chest infection. Denise had a viral infection which affected her ears and head. Alison had labyrinthitis. Mike had sore throats. All of them describe the onset in similar terms, using almost the same words, describing both the tiredness which 'dragged on' and the fact that they were 'knocked out'. As Lizzie says:

◈ It was June, maybe May. I got a virus which everybody got at the time and I just didn't pick up. It knocked me.

The most vivid account of a sudden onset is given by the GP, Alistair:

◈ I remember its onset very dramatically because I'd just run the Glasgow marathon about a week before. We were on our way to our timeshare in the Lake District. I was driving down the Kirkstone Pass, just past Ambleside, and suddenly I felt like I'd been hit by a flu bug. I mean, halfway down, just 'bam', cold and shivery, and when we got out of the car I had to sit down after 15 feet. I completely lost the power of my legs and that's how they stayed for the next three or four years.

His case is atypical because he is adamant that there was no concurrent infection:

◈ All I know is that my ME, and one or two others that I've read about, have come on with no viruses involved at all … I think it's just something that happened.

Two men and two women describe the onset of ME as gradual. Listening to them talking, however, I am not totally convinced that their experiences are so different from those of others who describe the onset as sudden. Their reporting may be related to their previous experience of health and illness. Possibly a very active past and rugged well-being makes some people oblivious or resistant to the early signs that something is wrong, to what seems to them an unlikely possibility of ill health. Three people felt ill for a year or more yet struggled on until a dramatic heightening of symptoms forced them to stop. Jamie, who describes his onset as gradual, says he felt unwell but 'just ignored all these things, and I tended, when put under pressure, to just work all the harder.' Janet also describes the onset of ME as gradual. But she is the wife of a busy GP with four small children, who could not stop – someone in different circumstances probably would have done. She describes four bouts of bad flu, getting up out of her bed from each one 'to start my life again and resume my duties'. Finally, there was no carrying on:

◆ I couldn't read, I couldn't do anything except listen to the radio and that's all I did for the best part of two years.

But, Phil, who describes his onset as sudden, tells a story which is very similar. Over the course of a year he admits he was overdoing things by trying to keep going in a very stressful job, despite feeling exhausted and being very vulnerable to infections. He admits that there were warning signs, then:

◆ **One day I woke up aware that something had happened.**

The 'something' was the start of an illness which so far has lasted for twelve years.

Ray may be the genuine exception to a sudden onset, but possibly he was also the most fit and the most oblivious to ill health. He describes a childhood in which he had an unusually high pain threshold:

◆ **I had boils in my ears and I never even knew they were there.**

This is a man who is a stranger to illness and pain. His description of the onset of ME as gradual is convincing, yet even he admits that his family noticed something was wrong before he did:

◆ **I just started feeling a bit tired. It never hit me like a tidal wave. I was never one to go to the doctor. I never had a sick day off in my life. It was my family who picked up on how hard I was working.**

But after a year he had to admit that he was 'going downhill'. Now, with the wisdom of hindsight, Ray looks back on that year of malaise and says:

◆ **The foolish bit is that I never looked into it. I never looked into ME at all. Not until a few months ago. I never knew anything about it.**

So, did Ray have a mild form of ME from the beginning? Or, exactly like Phil, did he push himself beyond his limits until a post-viral illness became ME? Unfortunately, we can only speculate, and guess.

Finally, May says that there was no sudden onset, nor can she recall any infection. She describes her illness mostly in terms of feeling depressed and exhausted. She recalls:

⬦ Complete and utter tiredness, no energy, no appetite and sitting around the house, sleeping 12–14 hours a day.

She also says, perhaps significantly:

⬦ I did not see any purpose in life.

Did she have the same illness as the others, or is she one of the 10–15 per cent who, according to Shepherd, are suffering from a psychiatric illness? It is impossible to judge.

Onset among young people

For the young people it is much harder to tell how and when ME begins. Most of them report a long history of feeling unwell or permanently tired while carrying on at school. If they felt ill from a young age, they had no baseline of good health which would have enabled them to report that something was wrong. Feeling worn out and not having the same energy levels as their peers was their norm. They knew no different, nor could they articulate the onset of an unfamiliar malaise.

The account given by the majority of the young people is of years of feeling utterly drained by school before a major relapse forced them to stop altogether. There is a fairly consistent picture of children struggling on at school, never well, but without anyone linking the exhaustion to illness. David's mother says that he was probably ill from the age of 7 when he was off school for a year with a series of viral illnesses. He always found school hard going. Then, when he was 14, he suffered a major relapse from which he has never recovered. The story is almost identical for Josh. Kirsty had sore throats and viral infections until, like David and Josh, she crashed at the age of 15. Jessie had two years of pain and tiredness with undiagnosed appendix problems, until:

◆ I got a virus and it just completely knocked me out and I don't think I was back in school full-time ever again.

Rachel and Ruby both remember a sudden start to their illness following a viral infection. Ruby's mother recalls her daughter picking up flu from the GP's surgery and not re-covering. Flu developed into glandular fever, and glandular fever progressed to ME. These are anecdotal case histories, but until we have a study of prevalence, we have no other evidence.

For two of the young people in my sample there may have been precipitating factors other than infection. Chris questions whether the onset of the symptoms which developed into ME was related to working with animals. He, like the others, recalls becoming ill with a virus, but it was at a time when he was working with pigs:

◆ When I became ill I was working at the Agricultural School with the pigs. So I was working with the pigs at the time, and

**my knees were covered with grease for handling the pigs
and I was eating my sandwiches and it was only days after
I became ill. I remember there were black finger marks on
my bread. And then I became ill.**

Was Chris exposed to something which, combined with a
viral infection, triggered his long illness? Were his greasy
sandwiches a factor in the development of ME? We don't
know. But Chris is not the only one to link ME to possible
exposure to chemicals. Alison became ill after she treated
children at school with lindane for head lice. Again, there
is no proof, but the hypothesis that ME can be triggered by
exposure to toxins and chemicals has support in the findings of some research papers.[13]

Stress as a trigger

It is not clear what role stress plays in the onset, or indeed the
progression, of ME. Evidence is mostly anecdotal, and
it is not useful to draw general conclusions from individual
case histories. Some people report that they were under
unusual stress at the time when they became ill, but others do
not. And for every person who becomes ill with ME during or
immediately following a stressful period in their lives, there are
thousands who are just as upset, overworked and strained who
do not. One of the problems here is the meaning of the word
'stress' – it has become so stretched and overworked that adver-
tisers use it to sell everything from tea to scented candles; similarly, primary school children have adopted the term to
describe their feelings about tests or broken relationships.[14]

But there are degrees of stress. There is a world of difference between feeling overworked and tired for a limited period, and being exposed to chronic, severe physical or mental strain and pressure. Unrelenting stress from which there is no escape, or a life crisis, or a shock event such as an accident are thought to be factors which might push some people into ME, especially if they battle on rather than stopping to let their bodies recover. Shepherd concludes, 'It could well be that repeated episodes of acute stress or prolonged periods of stress are important risk factors in the development of ME/CFS. High levels of stress certainly seem to have a very negative impact on the chances of recovering from ME/CFS.'[15]

There seem to be two separate questions here. First, is prolonged or acute stress a precipitating factor in the onset of ME? Second, does struggling on when physically and mentally burnt out prevent us from recovering from what might otherwise be a self-limiting, post-viral fatigue state and push us into full-blown ME? While there is some evidence that stress may play a role in both the onset and development of ME, as yet we do not understand either the processes or mechanisms involved, nor why some people can ride the storm and recover, while others become chronically disabled.

Among the people I talked to, some – but by no means all – reported high levels of stress at the time of developing ME. Those who were stressed and who started to feel tired and unwell, carried on working in demanding jobs or fulfilling heavy domestic roles when probably they should have stopped. We should not be surprised that people do battle on. Our society praises and rewards those who are seen to work hard and play hard, and to be permanently on the go. We are a 24-hour culture. People in the UK work longer hours than anywhere else in Europe. The media loves to report the achievements of those who manage to squeeze several lives into one, and to praise women who combine high-powered jobs with mothering. Our role models are often people who are able to burn candles at both ends. We are all of us under pressure to be busy, busy, busy.

Of the seven women in my sample, three said that they were under stress when they first started to feel ill. If I had asked a random sample of seven women without ME if their lives were stressed, I wonder whether the outcome would have been any different? From my small sample, I cannot draw any general conclusions. Were the stress levels amongst the women simply representative of the population as a whole or a significant co-factor with the onset of ME? Janet said that she was overstretched looking after four young children as well as fulfilling what she referred to as 'all her duties' as the wife of a GP in a rural practice. May reports long-term stress caused by the financial worries and the physical strain of running a newsagent's business. Lizzie began her university course in a state she describes as burn out:

◈ I had had a very rough time doing my A levels ... it was rough because I wasn't good at managing my stress levels and so I was absolutely exhausted. When I started university, I couldn't put pen to paper. I felt completely full up and I needed time off.

In contrast, Chloe and Fiona were fit, happy and fulfilled. Far from being stressed, these women talk about the pleasure and fun they were getting from their lives. Chloe says, 'I led a very active life and I enjoyed it.' Fiona says, 'Life was good.' Denise also says she was not particularly stressed, although her father had died two years previously. Alison, recently back from six months in Tibet, had bought herself a cello and was planning more trips abroad. Stress was not part of the picture.

Five of the seven men in my sample describe their lives as stressed – particularly at work – when the first signs of illness began. But this is not unusual, nor out of line for the general population. A recent study of work-related stress suggests that five million workers in the UK now have very high levels of occupational stress[16] – but not all of these go on to develop ME. Ray and Phil describe their stress levels as very high. Ray was under immense pressure as he juggled his job as a car mechanic with setting up his own business, with racing at weekends, while Phil tried to do the jobs of two people, commuting between Glasgow and Edinburgh. Jamie says he was stressed, overworking, doing too much. Mike says he was stressed at work and pressurised by deadlines. Liam talks a lot about stress but also questions its role in the onset of his illness. Prior to becoming ill he was trying to build up a university department which was run down and not doing any significant research, while at the same time he was supervising the building of a new family house. His mother had died two years earlier and his father had re-married. Asked about the link between stress levels and the onset of ME, he is reluctant, without diagnostic evidence, to draw any conclusions.

The remaining two men reject the idea of a stress-related onset. The only possible contributory factor might have been the tough physical workouts which they both regularly put themselves through, Fraser on the rugby pitch and Alistair running marathons. However, Fraser shakes his head at the possibility of this influencing the onset of his illness:

◆ I was probably at my physical peak. I was never expecting
   anything like this to come along.

Alistair does not commit himself either way, considering the role of physical overexertion a possible but weak hypothesis:

◆ I just wonder how much having trained for this marathon …
   how much I exhausted my system. I don't know. I'd run six
   or seven marathons before with no bother at all. I don't
   know. I put it down literally to what I call 'GAK'. God Alone
   Knows. It's a mystery.

Stress among young people

The concept of stress as a contributory factor for the young people is a different matter altogether. Once they start to feel even slightly unwell, children and adolescents must find school a nightmare, yet they carry on either because that is what is expected of them, or because without a baseline of well-being they do not understand that school should not feel this bad.

None of the young people report any specific incident which was more stressful than usual prior to the onset of symptoms. There were no major life events for any of them. Mostly the young people talk about the stress of coping with school once they became ill; they do not talk about being stressed by school or unhappy while they were still fit. Ruby says she 'had lots and lots of friends in school'. Kirsty loved school, although as she became increasingly unwell it drained more and more of her energy. She describes the last years as:

◆ **Exceptionally difficult. Even carrying a bag. Even that, little things like that, was really a struggle.**

Rachel pours scorn on the diagnosis that she was afraid of school rather than ill:

◆ **Afraid of school? But why am I still wanting to go?**

Speaking for all the young people, she makes the crucial point about difficulties at school being the result of being ill, not the other way round:

◆ **I think I did turn slightly school phobic at one point but it wasn't because I didn't like school; it was because of what was happening to me. I couldn't cope with school. I just couldn't process the information. I didn't have friends because it was just too much.**

We have to listen to Rachel and believe her. Of course, school is a source of stress if you are feeling ill. And for some of the young people, like David and Josh, there are no memories of school without illness because they became ill when they were too young to alert adults and persuade them to react appropriately.

Stress and illness are inextricably linked for the young people who persevere at school or at university. They are trying to achieve what normal young people achieve with half, a quarter or a tenth of the physical, mental and emotional resources. They are courageous, but all of them pay dearly for their years of stoicism.

CHAPTER 2

Telling it how it is

The interview subgroup felt that CFS brought their lives
to a standstill, completely disrupted all aspects of their
pre-illness lifestyle, and ravaged their sense of self. The
impact of CFS on their lives was so total and devastating
that participants had considerable difficulty accepting the
illness and its consequences.
ANDERSON AND FERRANS [1]

Most descriptions of ME miss the essence of it and fall short
of capturing its reality. Part of the problem is the word
'fatigue'. It is both a red herring and a hopelessly inadequate
description of how people feel. Although ME sufferers are
drained and exhausted to the core, they are not tired in a
floppy, nice-to-have-a-nap kind of way, such as after a bout
of flu when bed feels good and snuggling under the covers
for a few days brings a gradual return to well-being. ME
is a total exhaustion of body and mind; a nerve-jangling,
twitchy, overstretched and overwrought kind of tiredness
which cannot be relieved by rest or sleep. It is as if someone
has frayed the ends of every nerve in the body and left them
raw and exposed. It brings an overwhelming need to close
down sensory input and, for many, to retreat from ordinary
everyday stressors – conversation, noise, light, movement,
TV – since they are agonising to deal with. Everyone said
that they were *not* fatigued; they were catastrophically
overstretched. The inability to find words to describe ME
is a leitmotif through the transcripts. Some describe the

tired-but-wired sensation as ongoing jet lag, or the first day after a general anaesthetic, or 'a system closed down'. Some say they feel poisoned in every single cell of their bodies.

A better way to describe ME is 'running on empty' but the simile is only a partial description since no one knows exactly what has run out.[2] People who have ME are like cars with no petrol or oil, and no garage in sight where they can be topped up. They are trying to run the complex machinery of their bodies and minds without some vital lubricant which makes them go. ME feels like living on a tiny trickle of energy instead of a full flow. This feeble drip-feed drastically limits the activity of body, mind and emotions. When the trickle runs dry, it is necessary to stop to avoid further damage. So when they try to achieve more than their trickle of energy can fuel, they hurt themselves further, exacerbating symptoms and risking relapse.

Everyone in the survey said it is impossible to convey what ME feels like. They struggled to find words so that others could understand and empathise. Jamie, a fluent, articulate man, a writer and storyteller, ground to a halt several times as he tried to describe his illness:

◆ My world just collapsed, you know. My interpretation of it afterwards was that it was like a system closed down ... Jesus. I don't know. It's a ... well it's so many different things, but basically it's a crippling illness. It's left me with ... well I don't know what it's left me with.

Despite being a seasoned campaigner on behalf of people with ME, Marilyn too said she had great difficulties explaining ME to others. Referring to a woman at her work-place (and we all know this woman!), she said:

◆ Do you know, I have this problem? This person cannot
understand what ME is. She thinks it's all in the mind. I
didn't know where to start with it so I shut up. I just did
not know how to explain it to her. I can't get it across.
It's so unique.

Tired but wired: the hyper-crash cycle

To me, ME feels like being in a state of constant 'fright and flight'. Imagine being shocked by unexpected bad news. The heart pounds, we breathe quickly and shallowly, our muscles tense up, we shake, we go hot and cold, our faces turn ashen and our minds go blank. If you ask someone in a state of shock, perhaps following an accident or after terrible news about a loved one, to resume their concentration on some-thing which needs management and organisation, they cannot. This is how people with ME feel much of the time. In the early stages of the illness, and in severe cases, this is the normal bodily state. Later, as a slow recovery begins, it is possible to tolerate slightly more, and then slightly more again. But it is a long slow business.

When my teenage son relapsed severely, he started to pour sweat. He soaked the bed nightly. He poured sweat just living. Getting out of bed and having a shower soaked him in more ways than one. To compensate for lost fluid, he had to keep drinking (go to a meeting of ME people and you will see that most of them clutch bottles of water). This went on for two years. Any physical, intellectual or emotional exertion such as answering the phone would produce a racing heart (which I could feel heaving through his T-shirt), shaking, trembling and sweating. His body was shouting out to be left alone. Now, four years down the line, the sweating and the need to drink water returns at low points in his diurnal rhythm, or when he pushes himself too much or is forced into a situation over which he has no control. (Or when he watches Manchester United on TV – I know he is getting better because the other night he watched a whole football match with only a slightly wet T-shirt by the time the final whistle went.) This is not fatigue. This is a state of overstimulation which results in near or total collapse.

'One of the things which has been shown over and over again in people with fibromyalgia and Chronic Fatigue Syndrome is that biologically, they have an inability to respond appropriately to stressors.'[3] When laboratory animals are continuously exposed to stressors such as toxic substances, extreme heat and cold, loud noises and electrical shocks, in the end their adrenal glands become overstimulated, their lymphatic organs shrink, they lose weight, they develop ulcers and they die. Although ME is sometimes described as a stress-related illness, what stress means in this context is 'the non-specific response of the body to any demand.'[4] So, while healthy people cope with the demands which assault their senses, responding appropriately to what is relevant while ignoring what is not, people with ME have lost the ability to manage the sensory input of their environment. Dr

Bell's suggestion of 'The Mall Test' as a way of differentiating those who have ME from those who do not is spot-on.[5] Anyone who walks into a busy shopping precinct and is still standing after 10 minutes almost certainly does not have ME. Schools, shopping malls, large stores, cafes, hospital waiting rooms and corridors, cinema foyers and supermarkets are all environments in which people are bombarded by visual and aural input over which they have little or no control. Each context is a nightmare of sensory overload. Being exposed to such ordinary demands of living often results in a worsening of symptoms and may lead to relapse.

Early into my own relapse, I was admitted to hospital because my GP suspected meningitis. At that time I was extremely vulnerable to sensory input and needed to be left alone in a quiet, familiar, predictable environment. Instead, I was admitted to a neurological ward. The input was pure, exquisite agony, increasing with every hour. I tried to block out some of the noise and light by drawing the curtains round my bed (which were always pulled open again), by hiding my head under the pillows, by closing my eyes. By 'visiting time' I was shaking all over, my mouth was parched and I was drinking litre after litre of water – a sure sign that my body was distressed. I knew I was in deep trouble and my nervous system could not take much more. Finally, I could not lie or sit still. I walked the corridors, left the ward, climbed stairs. If a body could scream, mine would have done. The hospital staff thought I was mad. But this was not a panic attack – I was not worried, anxious or frightened. It was physical not emotional trauma. My body was trying, and failing, to cope with an overwhelming environment, and at some fundamental, chemical level things were becoming wildly out of kilter. In the end, I phoned my husband to tell him to get me out. And while I waited, I had to keep moving, pacing up and down, and clawing the walls, despite complete exhaustion. I felt as if my body was a vase which had cracked all over and was about to fall into a thousand fragments. Although from the outside I looked hysterical, it was my body not my mind which was stressed to a degree which was intolerable. I don't know what would have happened if I had not got out of there.

While I was writing this chapter, I received the following e-mail from Ciara MacLaverty, who has been ill since 1987. It is painful to read, and offers no happy ending, but it captures the essence of what it feels like to have ME.

◆ I am confined to bed for 80–95 per cent of my day and often when I make any degree of effort, however small (e.g., getting up, going for a short walk, talking on the phone) within minutes my body often gears up into what I term 'the hyper'. The 'hyper' is like a full-blown panic attack without the psychological element. I am **not** frightened or nervous in any way but my body becomes both taut and shaky; waves of prickly sweat run from the soles of my feet to my scalp; my mind suddenly becomes less 'brain fogged' and my thoughts race and jump about. I feel ransacked by adrenaline, yet profoundly weak. It is as if my nervous system is going into crisis mode in a desperate attempt to process everyday information such as polite conversation or the layout of an unfamiliar room.

An average one- or two-hour 'hyper' can take two to twenty-four hours to come down from and invariably causes me insomnia. I can take tranquillisers *and* sleeping pills after seeing friends for a couple of hours in the evening and still only scrape four hours' sleep. 'Tired but wired' is a phrase I readily relate to.

During my relapse of the last two years, every 'hyper', without fail, has been followed by a 'crash', during which I feel as if I am a ninety-year-old woman who has just been injected with a cocktail of two parts horse tranquilliser to one part arsenic. My concentration drains away to the point where I can't read a page or watch TV. I feel as if there is not enough blood or oxygen in my brain … and there is nothing I can do but lie curled up in the foetal position with my eyes closed. Frequently there's a burning head and neck pain too. This 'crash' phase usually lasts several days – sometimes weeks. At such times there is simply no other option but to lie there and wait it out, avoiding as much stimulation as possible. The boredom, loneliness and the frustration are searing at this time and it takes great depths of inner resource just to get through. I don't sleep during the day, but drift in and out of sickly flu-like dozes. At night I revert to sleeping for nine or ten hours straight and wake feeling like I'm just coming round after a major operation.

I could remain in this 'crash' condition for weeks and months if I resigned myself to it, but invariably my spirits take a battering and I long to try to do *something*, so once again I try to build myself up slowly. I sit in a chair or have a friend to visit or take a short walk outside. I can 'get away' with these kinds of activity for a few days but inevitably, no matter how much I 'pace' myself and tip toe, the 'hyper' leaps out like a pantomime villain and the vicious cycle begins all over again.

What is wrong with my body that allows these agonising and exhausting swings? It is not a fear of situations that kick starts the 'hyper' symptoms, but the body's physical inability to provide the necessary energy – mental and physical.

This is exactly what it is like. People talk about how they crank themselves up to manage some trivial or minimal event such as spending an hour with a relative or friend. From the outside there are no obvious signs that all is not well, yet the façade of normality may be hiding an increasingly physically stressed state as ill people try to pass for normal, try to carry on talking and listening, try to keep walking, try to keep going. Healthy people do not see the bodies which are rapidly running out of steam, of oomph, of energy – of whatever allows normal people to lead their normal lives and not be instantly drained. After anything which feels like an effort (and the definition of 'an effort' can be anything from cutting up a lettuce or writing an e-mail to walking to the post office), it is often necessary to retreat to a quiet, silent, controlled world so that stretched, shaking bodies can return to something like a resting state. But these struggles to maintain an equilibrium of energy are invisible except to each person with ME and those very close to them.

Unpredictable

One of the most distinctive, and most difficult features of ME, is its fluctuating nature as the illness meanders along its course with often unpredictable ups and downs and plateaux. The most common long-term pattern is a very slow and gradual return to partial or near-complete recovery in a zig-zagging line of good, bad and indifferent health. Commonly, over the years, the highs gradually get higher and longer, and the lows not so long-lasting or deep. The most common scenario is that people spend years of their lives on a roller-coaster of ups and downs, doing a bit too much or just doing what they normally do, experiencing an intensification of symptoms – sometimes for a reason, but not always – resting until they feel better, then getting back on the ride again. They mostly work and play somewhere between the world of the well and the world of the sick, belonging in neither. Only a small proportion of people make the complete crossing back into their former lives.[6, 7, 8, 9, 10] The lack of control over the course of the illness, together with the fact that they do not know when or if it will end, means that people with ME do not have a lifestyle so much as life-chaos.

Among my sample, eight out of the fourteen adults have achieved a lasting recovery of between 80 per cent and 100 per cent of their previous fitness; three now function at about 50 per cent; three are only 40 per cent recovered after many years. The course of the illness for the young people is more disappointing than for the adults. Of the seven young people interviewed, two have achieved a 70–80 per cent recovery; the rest rate their present level of disability as

50–80 per cent. Those who remain ill continue to experience the same fluctuations in symptom level and the same variation in their ability to function from day to day, week to week.

The ups and downs of ME inform and dominate their lives as people try to work out what they dare to do right now, tomorrow or next week. As Alison says, she has to wait until she opens her eyes in the morning and runs a quick physical check-up before she can guess at her energy levels, and then not always accurately:

◆ I woke up and felt OK. I got out of bed and went to get breakfast and suddenly all my energy was gone. It was just urghhh ... collapse. I went back to bed. After a bit I felt OK again so I got up and went into the next room to do some small task and again suddenly complete collapse and feeling terrible. I just can't predict from one half hour to the next what I am going to feel like.

The unpredictability of symptoms means that in the short term there is no forward planning – and this means not knowing the day before, and sometimes even the hour before, whether it is possible to fulfil an engagement, go for a walk, risk a trip to the shops or even get out of bed. Everything has to be done on the instant. Even in its mild to moderate form, ME brings symptoms which are neither stable nor predictable, as Fiona describes:

◆ My main symptom was great fatigue. I would be OK for two or three days and think: 'Great. I've got over it.' And then hit a low. I would feel the colour going right out of my face, a cold feeling. I'd think: 'Oh,' and have to sit down and very often I'd go to sleep. It was a horrible feeling. It took away all spontaneity. You couldn't plan anything because you'd think: 'I can do that' and then: 'Well, just how am I going to do that?' It had a tremendous effect on normal life. It just was not predictable.

Many healthy people fail to understand this unpredictability, perhaps judging those with ME as unreliable free spirits because they cancel appointments time after time, not understanding that this invisible part of ME is beyond anyone's control. Living with ME is like living with a cruelly erratic presence. But in time, and to some extent, one can learn to read the signs and beat it at its own game. It is possible, as these transcripts show, to get on top of the ups and downs and to find some stability. It means tuning in to small signs of fading energy and knowing when to stop. People become skilled at this survival game, and by keeping a weather eye on symptom levels, they can live a more 'normal' life. Psychiatrists call this 'maladaptive behaviour', but wisdom and self-preservation are more useful and realistic terms.

Relapse

Most people with ME come to accept the ups and downs and the variation in symptom levels within parameters which they have set themselves. It's like having a thermometer which registers an acceptable minimum and maximum level of functioning. Even if they feel ill, tired or wretched, so long as they can manage to keep going, so long as they can get up the next day and start again, then life is to some extent under their control and to a degree tolerable. But sometimes, catastrophically, this system fails.

The very worst thing that can happen is that we slip off this narrow path of existence and start to plummet down-hill. To contemplate a full-blown relapse is to despair. How could one endure it a second time, or a third? Yet some people have to because of the fickle, unpredictable nature of the illness. As Ciara MacLaverty describes:

◆ The dominating emotion in the first months of my massive second relapse was one of disbelief. Having lived with the illness for eleven years, I was extremely dubious about my chances of ever making a full recovery, but after being stable for eight years, I possessed an innate confidence that I would, at least, never get any worse. The symptoms and I had fallen into a grudging truce. The ME was my elephant in the living room. I tripped over it and routinely got squashed and thoroughly inconvenienced by it, but I had managed to live a life in and around it.

All that changed suddenly on Midsummer's Day, 1998. How was I to know that it would be the last day of my limited but cherished freedom? I returned from an open-air pop festival with signs of a summer cold. The 'bug' passed within a day or two, but in its wake I felt the 'poisoned heavy fatigue' on a scale that I hadn't felt for years. It shocked and frightened me, but I kept hoping and believing it would pass, until weeks turned into months and it became agonisingly clear that, yet again, some biological catastrophe had occurred.

How I railed against it. I tried every remedy I could think off, every 'coping strategy'. I remember dragging myself out of bed, sweating and shaking across the street to my local park in the hope that the fresh air would help. It was a crisp autumn day and when I looked at the leaves I could only think of all the autumns before – three bedbound autumns in the 1980s, followed by happier, progressively more active autumns in the 1990s. And now, as the leaves fell once more, I was catapulted back into the living nightmare. One of the hardest aspects of ME to live with is not only the fact that time doesn't always heal. It's the devastating realisation that time can make you worse again.

There are no satisfactory explanations for these terrible crashes. Anecdotal evidence suggests that the risk factors are overdoing it (and there is no formula for calculating that one), a viral infection or an increase of stress and pressure. Or all three. Sometimes a crash comes out of the blue – reducing its victim to rubble. For those who have had ME in its severe form, and who have climbed partially out of the pit, warning signs of a slide back into severe ill health strike a note of terror. They know what it is like, and they don't want to go back there ever again. They hope and pray that the return of the symptoms is anything other than ME back in full, relentless force.

But it happens. Like Ciara, some people achieve a partial recovery, perhaps reaching 70 per cent or 80 per cent of their former energy level, only to suffer a major relapse. This is what happened to me when I returned to full-time work after seven years. I was never really well, always balancing my activities so that I managed two-thirds of each day, and rested for one-third. But after the agony of full-blown ME for three years, this was acceptable. I decided to return to work, commuting to Glasgow where I plunged into a hefty research project which would have challenged even the physically and mentally robust. But I was never right. Most evenings were spent lying on the sofa, and weekends were burn-out. I made excuses for not joining in the evening outings with my colleagues to the pub or ten-pin bowling. How could I explain? I did the fieldwork, wrote the papers. My colleagues saw the surface of my existence but not its sick underbelly. Finally, I collapsed – big time. I cannot put into words my despair as I was forced to face the fact that ME had returned.

For many, the long years of a half-life or quarter-life with ME are bad enough. The snail-pace crawl back to moderate health takes so long, and absorbs considerable quantities of energy, ingenuity, planning and lateral thinking. Along the way, ambitions, careers, hopes, plans, family and friends are cast off – but still this is for the most part bearable. In comparison, the possibility of losing that modicum of control and a fragile stability is unthinkable. A major relapse following partial or complete recovery is when we stop living all over again.

The legacy

Everyone asks, 'Will I get better? When will I get better?' Chloe, having realistically given up any hope of a short term or sudden recovery, does what many do – a yearly reckoning:

◆ It's every Christmas or New Year I think: 'Right, next year
   I'm going to be well and I want to be well', and every
   Christmas and New Year comes ... and, yes, I'm slightly
   better, but ... [she trails off in tears] ... It's been five years.
   I would just hate somebody to tell me, 'Another five years
   and you're still going to have it', because I feel then I would
   have ended it. I can't think I'm going to go through another
   five years of this. I just don't want to go through another
   five years. You wouldn't wish this on your worst enemy.

Nor is a future-imperfect the preserve of the still-sick. ME
also leaves its imprint on those who are fully, or almost fully,
recovered. What is left behind may be an inability to reach
the sort of fitness that existed before the illness, or a nagging
return of cognitive problems, or something more elusive – a
waiting and watching when flu-like symptoms occasionally
return with stress or a viral infection. Liam admits he has
never fully recovered:

◆ I'm totally exhausted on a Saturday. Sometimes I'm in a
   vegetative state and I can hardly string words together.

Today, fifteen years after onset, Liam still cannot follow his
passion for music. He rarely risks a concert in case the
volume of sound or a sudden crash of drums brings a return
of the painful brain sensations which continue to dog him.
   For others too there is a residue of physical or cognitive
or emotional disability. Mike remains about 10 per cent
disabled:

◆ I may look like I'm fully fit, but when it actually comes to doing anything that's a bit more strenuous, then no, I'm not able to do it. It's not because I'm physically unfit, it's because my body won't let me.

The further people have moved from the illness, the paler is the colour of the fear, but no one said it had really gone. Liam and Fraser both talk about an 'unease'. Fraser feels physically recovered, but:

◆ There is a wee mental thing still left in there without a doubt … when you get a fair wallop with the flu it's quite a shock to the system, so I think there's a wee bit left in there, a wee seed of doubt as to whether something might happen again in the future.

Alistair talks of a fear that accompanies every new viral infection:

◆ I think it's 95 per cent behind me. But I still get the odd days; I mean all last week I was feeling what I call not ill but not well. The trouble is, having had ME, you're far more sensitive about diagnosing yourself, and whether it's just a normal virus, you immediately go into panic mode: Is this it again? I got a flu thing at Christmas which wasn't bad enough to be off work, but it took more time than usual to clear and I thought: 'Oh Jesus, here we go again'.

May talks about a watchfulness that never quite goes away:

◆ Once you have had it, I don't think you get totally clear
of it. I think you're always prone to having some kind of
relapse to a greater or lesser degree. I think you learn to live
with it and you start to recognise the symptoms earlier and
you stand back and say, 'Right, time to reassess'.

Emily calls it a legacy:

◆ There's a legacy. There is a definite legacy. I suspect there'll
always be a legacy. I'm sure about that, but I can't be sure
whether or not it's finished. All I know is that there has
been a long interval, but when the long interval becomes
the cessation, you never know. And we shall never know.

And so it is for almost everyone. ME leaves its invisible foot-
print in a weakened immune system, in the brain chemistry,
in the circuitry of hormones, in the central nervous system
and in the psyche. Probably the most terrifying thing about
ME is that often there is no absolute ending. Josh's father,
Nelson, has gone through fire and brimstone and still he
does not know if the final curtain is at last coming down on
twelve years of anguish:

◆ Josh has started to make some real progress this summer.
I find myself writing as if the worst is past and we have
survived. But of course, like everything else with ME, we
don't know. But if we didn't believe that … then we would
probably be sunk.

CHAPTER 3

How bad can it get?

Suffice it to say, 'What life?' I was existing. I wasn't living.
MAY

In polite chat I often tell people that 'I'm having a bad
patch', but if I'm honest I've been completely unable to
spend more than two hours out of bed a day for the past
three years and I've never felt well, even for a single day,
in the past fifteen years. This is the horrible reality that I
don't throw into polite or everyday conversation.
CIARA MACLAVERTY

Using the self-rating ME Disability Scale[1], the people in my
study scored a mean of 77 per cent disability at their worst.
The adults in the California self-help group were sicker than
those in Scotland with a mean disability level of 83 per cent
at their lowest point compared with 68 per cent for the UK
adults. The young people were sicker still; their mean disability level was 94 per cent at their worst. This relationship
does not change when current disability levels are reported.
The mean disability level now for all subjects is 38 per cent.
For UK adults it is 26 per cent compared with 53 per cent for
the group in California. The young people remain on
average 56 per cent disabled today.

In my sample, the severity of symptoms and degree of
disability varied considerably. At one end of the continuum
are Fraser and Alistair who rated themselves as 40 per cent

disabled at their lowest point, and who have gone on to make a full recovery over a period of five and six years respectively. Ian, Fiona, Liam, May and Bruce Campbell were ill for only two years before making a substantial recovery. At the other end of the spectrum are Denise, Alison, Chloe and Phil who remain 50–60 per cent disabled after many years. The young people as a group are more disabled than the adults and are recovering much more slowly. Two rated themselves 75–80 per cent disabled, and five 100 per cent disabled, at their worst. None have recovered more than 30 per cent of their former level of fitness and four remain more than 50 per cent disabled after an average of ten years.

Fraser was able to carry on working as a firefighter throughout his illness, although he had to give up rugby training and found that life was reduced to work, walking the dog and lying on the sofa. Alistair kept working as a GP, despite the fact that on many days he felt 'hellish'. Both classify themselves as 'mild to moderate' cases, and both use the terms 'lucky' and 'fortunate' in their interviews, acknowledging their awareness of others who are much more severely affected. Lizzie describes a typically moderate level of illness when she says:

◆ I didn't have severe pain. I had like a vice around my head. It felt tight. I would get up in the morning and would go, 'Right, today I'm going to look for a job,' and I'd be excited, then about half an hour later I would be totally exhausted. I'd be so depressed because I'd be like that for the rest of the day.

In contrast, Janet, May, Phil, Alison, Jamie and Denise were so ill that they were bedbound, housebound and barely able to function. Phil had to return to his parents to be looked after. Alison had to retreat to a Buddhist monastery.

The following, from a scientist who has been getting progressively more ill for twenty years, arrived while I was writing this book, and captures sensitively and movingly both the severity and the nature of the illness:

◆ One of the things I recognise about my own situation is how all of my efforts here at home mask the seriousness of my own health. It is so clearly visible on holiday, especially the physical disability and I don't just mean the wheelchairs at the airports or the skeletal image cast on an Andalusian beach. There was the mental anguish of the recognition that I am not able to walk anywhere. This affected me far more than I would have imagined. Sitting there in the little hill towns of Andalusia, I was stuck to a seat outside a cafe as my 77-year-old mother-in-law and my wife wandered the little streets and looked over historical sites of interest. It is simply that one oozes sickness and dysfunction and that one is not part of normal society. One is sicker than other disabled persons lying about on the beaches or being wheeled about in airports, persons who can usually propel their own wheelchairs or who can enjoy the full spectrum of pleasure afforded by the Andalusian sunshine once they get there. I am more like an old infirm person than the semblance of any other physically disabled being.
Working here at home one covers over the cracks in one's predicament but on holiday there is nowhere to hide.

It is so important to record accurately, and in the words of sufferers, how severe symptoms can be. Phil gives the following account of the severity of his illness:

◆ My mind was blurred like mince. I was cognitively challenged and couldn't think straight. I was struggling to remember simple things like my own name, my flatmate's name, where I had to drive to get to work or whatever. My mind was just a complete blur. My limbs were very, very weak. That's what I remember more than anything, barely being able to stand. The analogy I have is like the newly-born calf or lamb, really struggling to find my feet. I remember fever, a sort of low-grade fever. I remember waking every night in this horrible sweat with a high temperature and a lot of achiness in my muscles. Also for the first time in my life there was a high-pitched whining in my ears, tinnitus. It felt well beyond flu. It felt more severe than any infection I have ever had in my life.

Symptoms as severe as these extend well beyond physical pain and disability, and disrupt any attempt to live a normal life. Because there is impairment at every level of functioning, people like Phil are consigned to a life of solitude and inactivity. He talks about being too ill to cope even with brief visits from his mates.

◆ I was living at my mum and dad's. They would usher them in, stay half an hour, sometimes in a darkened room, and usher them back out. I hated the visits. I felt almost like I was dying. I felt I was close to dying.

Severity in young people

Six of the seven young people were very seriously ill. I cannot draw any general conclusions from this sample about the severity of ME in children and young people compared with adults, nor can I say whether my sample is unusual in presenting the more extreme form of the illness. Possibly I came across these young people precisely because they were so ill and housebound, and were therefore linked to the local support network as a lifeline. No doubt others, less severely affected, are out there struggling through school or college, carrying on their education part-time, not severed from the society of their peers. But it is not rare for young people to become as ill as those in my sample.[2,3,4] Each of them knew of one or two others who were similarly affected. In telling their stories, I may be describing one end of the continuum of this disease. Others may feel as bad as this for a shorter time before starting to recover. Some may only experience some of the symptoms described, or they may experience the same symptoms but in a milder form. Far from diminishing the accounts reported here, an accurate description of the suffering endured by young people is one of the most important reasons for writing this book. It is crucial to record, recognise and acknowledge the catastrophic nature of ME and its impact on some young lives. While the media and the national ME association magazines tend to be dominated by stories of young people who do manage to carry on with their studies and with their social lives, accounts of those who are too ill to write about their quality of life are still not often seen or heard. As Josh says:

- There's all the difference in the world between functioning at 50 per cent and functioning at 20 per cent like me.

Yet doctors, the media and even the ME support groups tend to fight shy of such negative but honest accounts of ME, preferring the stories with happy endings to those of a never-changing, almost non-existent life. This may lead to the public being unaware of the extent and the severity of the illness. Kirsty told me:

- I was bedridden for between a year and a half, and paralysed for about six months or something like that. I just couldn't move at all on one side of my body.

Rachel spent thirteen months in hospital, first in a ward for children with infectious diseases, then in an adult HIV and Drug Rehab ward. At her lowest physical and emotional ebb, she felt she could not carry on:

- They would get me up and dressed because if you're not dead they get you up and dressed in hospital. It doesn't matter if you're going to die the next minute. I had about two tablespoons of Rice Krispies floating around in lots of milk and Dr W came in and I was just sitting there crying. Not for any particular reason, but I couldn't keep my head still or get my hand to my mouth so it was all down my front. Then I had to go on a NG tube because I was losing so much weight. It was so awful.

Rachel's health continued to deteriorate over a period of six years. With each inappropriate treatment or placement in an inappropriate institution, she became more ill. Finally, she cracked emotionally because her pain became unbearable:

> I was so ill and low. I don't think it was because it [my illness] was psychosomatic, it wasn't caused by my madness which they are trying to pin on me now, but I got to such a low point, I ended up cutting myself. It wasn't a suicide attempt. It was just ... I needed to do something.

Finally, here is Josh whose father describes his illness as a 'disaster':

> The worst thing about having ME, obviously, is having ME. It is spending three years in your bedroom looking at the walls, in pain, isolated, unable to read, write or talk with a brain like spaghetti. The worst thing is having a brain which no longer works and which I can't do anything about. It's like being in solitary confinement, except that I haven't done anything wrong.

CHAPTER **4**

Reaching parts other illnesses don't reach

As it constricts your capabilities, chronic illness does no
less than change your self-image and your personality.
Whoever you were before the diagnosis has already
metaphorically died.
KANE[1]

All the people in this study were, to varying degrees, physically, cognitively and emotionally disabled. Previously fit and healthy men and women experienced energy levels plummeting to zero. The change in physical fitness was often extreme with marathon-running, squash-playing macho men unable to walk a few yards without pain and exhaustion. Others were so cognitively impaired that they could not concentrate, absorb and process information, or speak in coherent sentences. Those who were previously calm and grounded individuals experienced mood swings and panic attacks. ME robbed people of their sense of self, their confidence and self-esteem. Individuals were affected in different ways – for some physical pain dominated while others hid from the ordinary input of the everyday world because their central nervous systems were so oversensitised.

The scope of potential symptoms makes doctors wary of ME. If each person who turned up in the surgery reported a headache, nausea and pain in the left ankle then doctors would be on more familiar territory. But the catalogue of symptoms – from paralysis to pain to panic attacks to constant infections to brain fog – vary from individual to individual, while many who are severely and chronically ill may cope with all these disabilities, and more.

Physical disability

When Alison bought *A Suitable Boy* by Vikram Seth, a novel of some 900 pages, she cut it into three pieces so that she could prop each chunk on the bed while she read. On bad days, Ruth crawls the short space from her studio room to the bathroom because her legs are too weak to carry her there. At her lowest point Fiona was too weak to hold up her head or brush her hair. In this study, these are the extreme cases. But even those with ME in its milder form sometimes experience the same destruction of fitness and physical health.

As a group, the men I interviewed were exceptionally fit prior to ME. Phil and Alistair ran marathons. Ray raced sports cars. Fraser trained as a rugby player. Mike went hill walking, taking his robust health for granted. These were active men, strangers to illness. Because they were so fit, being robbed of their stamina and strength was a bitter blow. No doubt there are those who would say that these men got off lightly. In fact they would agree, but the loss of physical health struck at the core of their self-perception. Before ME, they were fit macho men; after ME, they were men who walked the dog – slowly – and lay on the sofa. This is how Mike describes his physical condition:

◆ I suffered very bad myalgia in my legs. And there was the constant fatigue. I lived in a third-floor flat and I could only get up the stairs by resting on each landing. I used to be able to bound up two stairs at a time. Once in the flat, I wasn't going out. I was going out once a day and that was it.

It's not just the running around and training and working up a good sweat that these men have forfeited. It is the camaraderie of others that is a part of sport and team games. It is also a way of life which takes them outdoors, out into the fresh air, away from the pressure of their weekday jobs. Physical activity can push up our endorphin levels, making us feel good about ourselves, even euphoric. The men derived intense pleasure from getting out and working their bodies to a satisfied exhaustion. Their loss is significant. Mike considers himself 90 per cent better, but even now, he says with regret:

I don't even consider doing any sort of physical sport. I would really like more of an outdoor life. I don't want to be charging around running marathons, but I would just like to be able to get out and walk. I am always conscious of the fact that I can't go hill walking with someone. I'd be asking them to carry me back.

In my study, the men find the decline in their physical health more difficult to bear than the women. Not knowing when their fitness will return is intolerable. Fraser, a strapping big man, trained with commitment and passion as a rugby player before he became ill. The loss of his strength and stamina was harder to cope with than the pain and exhaustion. Listening to him talk, it is obvious how much it hurt. And how dumbfounded he was at the change:

It was a huge blow at the time. It knocked me down. When the penny actually dropped that I was physically unable to play – and I was getting to the age when I was at the peak of my powers – I knew this was taking it all away from me. A year would go by. A year and a half. And it was getting worse, you know, feeling: 'Christ, how long is this taking?' … If it had been a fracture or a torn ligament or whatever, someone would say, 'Fraser, right, in six months you'll be playing.' Or, 'In three months you'll be playing.' And that was fine. You knew how long you'd be off. But when I asked the doctors, 'How long do you think … ?' Well, how long is a piece of string? Nobody could tell me when it would come to an end. It was gnawing away all the time.

Fraser is the first to admit that his loss is nothing compared to the losses others suffer. But comparisons are odious; for him the loss of his exceptional fitness was a big issue. After four years, gradually and gingerly he did start playing rugby again.

But the women also report missing physical activity, although this is not their greatest loss, nor do they feel it as keenly as the men. They do not miss the competitive aspect of sport, the banter of their team-mates, nor, necessarily, pushing themselves to their limits. Their pleasure, they say, is getting out of the house and finding a quiet pleasure in walking alone or with friends in the fresh air. Only Chloe and Denise are similar to the men in the regret they express at giving up sporting activities. Chloe says:

I led a very active life and I enjoyed it. I was doing two step classes a week and swimming and I loved going out dancing.

Denise describes herself as 'a sporty person' prior to ME, and lists swimming, yoga, aerobics and line dancing as the things she most misses. Alison says jubilantly, 'I was going to climb mountains!' But, more typically, Janet talks of the solitary pleasure of walking. Asked what she considered her greatest loss, she replied:

 ◈ I used to lie in bed on a sunny day and wish I could be out walking. Every day that was bright I was really heartbroken that I couldn't be out enjoying it.

This is the bottom line. So many people with ME lie on their beds for months and years, looking out of the window, aware of wasting muscles, longing to be a part of the changing seasons rather than a passive onlooker.

Cognitive problems

OK, it is funny (for a while) when people put their keys away in the medicine cabinet and try to phone with the TV remote control and talk 'word salad'. Ray describes this state of mind as 'like I'm under water'. He tells stories of getting in the car and driving off on some particular errand only to come all the way back because he can't remember what the errand is. Or:

 ◈ I take the dog out and tie him to a railing to go into the shop, and he's beside you because you've not tied him up at all. You've gone through the motions but you've missed when you've been doing the knot and he's got up with a big knot on the end of his lead. This is just incredible.

More terrifying is the fact that long-established skills and abilities seem to vanish. Ray is appalled to find that he can no longer drive round the streets, let alone think about getting in a racing car:

⬦ My driving is shocking: hitting kerbs; wondering, maybe in a couple of months I'll have to make the decision to stop.

He tells his self-deprecating stories in a way that provokes laughter, but the laughter is not far from tears. It is not funny that competent individuals cannot drive or remember or read or solve problems or study. It is not funny that they cannot absorb information or make decisions or understand anything but the simplest instructions. Minds, once obedient and clear, are disobedient, cloudy and slow. The cogs don't turn. In his interview, Phil describes his brain as 'mincemeat'. Janet says she couldn't read for two years. Alison and her partner could not play the piano for seven years. Wells writes: 'For those of us, like myself, whose identity is based on our intellect and our achievements, the most frightening loss is that of our once sharp and dependable minds. Short-term memory problems and difficulty concentrating plague many of us. On a fairly good day I may forget a word. On a bad day I don't even have the ability to describe the word I've forgotten.'[2] The young people describe how difficult, sometimes impossible, it is to sit in a classroom with a mind that has seized up. They may appear stupid, they may be judged stupid, yet their intellectual ability is intact. The problems are to do with access, retrieval, memory and concentration. As Rachel explains:

◆ When you're listening, it goes in one ear and straight back out the other. I'm not thick. I would try and I would get good results but I would have to put in so much effort and no one would seem to realise it.

In a recent review of 20 papers relating to cognitive function, Shepherd concludes that all the authors' descriptions of intellectual disability falls short of the severity of symptoms reported by almost all his patients and that short-term memory problems are far worse than that implied in the diagnostic criteria for CFS.[3] People with ME are slow to acquire new information, slow to process any information and slow to cope with complex tasks. They find it difficult to take in information coming simultaneously from different sources, cannot do more than one thing at a time, and generally are unable to use their minds as they once did. In other words, cognitive disability is universally underplayed and underreported. Josh writes:

◆ My brain won't work. I tried studying today but I can't. Nothing goes in. I read the words and they bounce off. What can I do with myself? I'm going round the bend. It's been like this for four years.

Other studies show that cognitive impairment is a significant part of ME.[4,5,6,7] This is what most ME sufferers call 'brain fog'. The more ill and tired they are, the more their brains refuse to work. It is the mental equivalent of trying to map-read one's way through a peasouper of a fog, and is deeply frustrating and disabling. An inability to think clearly or easily probably affects at least two-thirds of ME sufferers.[8]

One day, some months into his illness, Liam was battling on with his university teaching. During a lecture he was giving, he caught himself using a term that was completely wrong. The experience shocked him:

◈ I realised when I thought about it that the word I had produced sounded similar but the meaning was totally different, at which stage I said that I wasn't going to lecture any more because I was in danger of producing utter nonsense. I mean, that stressed me.

He negotiated a term's sabbatical with the objective of writing up his research, but that too proved beyond him:

◈ I learned to operate a computer and all I was good for was tapping away at the keys. I mean, I was supposed to be writing articles. What I finished up doing was learning to work a computer and operate a word processing package.

This may sound enough of a challenge, but for Liam it was a mundane task which he performed at a low level. And even this exhausted him.

For those who use their minds to earn their living cognitive dysfunction can bring not only anxiety and frustration but also the threat of job loss, the end of a career and the destruction of self-confidence and self-identity. For people who rely on their intellectual abilities and who derive meaning and pleasure from their ability to think clearly and well, mental fog is a disaster. A thinker who cannot think is like a highly-trained athlete who loses the use of his legs. For four years following my relapse I experienced brain fog so severe that I could not write. Not even a shopping list. On many days, trying to write this project has been the mental equivalent of wading thigh deep through mud with weights on both legs. The inner monologue which previously accompanied me, making sense of things and giving meaning to experience, dried up.

Language problems

Embarking on an anthology of writing about the personal experience of CFIDS, Munsen writes of her potential contributors:

> As I culled submissions, writers with higher education degrees sent me notes apologising for their choppy sentences. Published poets told me the subject matter of their own illness was too painful, too difficult to convey. Reliable literary friends promised to write me pieces and then sent frantic e-mails saying they were bedbound, having a severe relapse, or too brain-fogged to begin. One writer – in a classic CFIDS haze – actually mailed me her medication schedule.[9]

The 'word-search engine' seems to go badly wrong for many people with ME. The ability to speak and write fluently can be crazily disrupted as people struggle to dredge up coherent sentences, stop half-way through a sentence, and substitute one word for another. Speaking, conversing and communicating, especially when exhaustion descends, is a daily problem. There are different kinds of substitutions – a word which starts with the same letter; a word with a similar meaning to the one intended; a word which sounds a bit like the one which was meant. Sometimes the words which pop out seem to have no relationship to the ones which were intended. Word salad replaces normal speech and friends and relations have to become interpreters. Alison talked about a 'swizzle chair', the 'nunks and muns' at the Buddhist centre, the 'decompression tablets' which her GP tried to prescribe, a 'pirate's carrot', and her 'nobility allowance' (which everyone deserves).

As I recover, I still struggle with language now. I remember an incident in California when I set off to introduce myself to the owner of a house that was to let. I knew her name was Estelle. I hadn't slept well the previous night and was deep in brain fog, managing to get lost several times during a simple, straight, quarter-mile walk from my place to hers. On the doorstep I actually said, 'Hello. I'm Estelle.' The mistake happened because I was trying so hard to remember her name, aware that my once razor-sharp memory was now a sieve through which words and ideas fell to earth never to be recovered. Still, it shocked me that I could be so brain-damaged, albeit temporarily, to do such a strange thing.

Liam describes his cognitive disability very much in terms of language impairment. Words and sentences became muddled. He used incorrect terminology. He found himself saying one thing when he meant another. He describes a trip to Hungary during his illness where he struggled to communicate with a foreign colleague. Instead of his usual quick replies to requests for English translations, Liam found himself floundering. He debates whether his problems with language reflect his general mental and physical exhaustion but concludes that this is not the case. More significantly, he also dismisses the idea that what he is experiencing is a simple word-search problem caused by memory loss. In front of a picture of a famous Roman sculpture of Romulus and Remus, he begins a sentence which tails off into nothing:

> 'Oh yes, that's the wolf that …' At that point I had a sinking feeling in my stomach and a sort of panic which told me not that I had forgotten the word, but that I no longer knew it. That's a totally different feeling. A feeling that something is on the tip of your tongue is uncomfortable, but a feeling that you don't know any longer is utter panic.

We can laugh at our ridiculous malapropisms but these language problems are significant both in their impact on everyday living and in differentiating ME from illnesses such as depression. Together with the cognitive difficulties of poor concentration and the effort required to deal with information, they suggest a dysfunctional brain. Studies on ME sufferers have found reduced blood flow in some areas of the brain, and Dr Shiela Bastien found IQ scores dramatically lowered in a group of educated people with ME, so much so that in some cases she describes their performances as 'startlingly close to the legal definition of idiocy.'[10]

Mood swings and loss of emotional control

It is not surprising that ME sufferers are sometimes emotional and upset as they struggle with the daily reality of a chronic, life-changing illness. At one end of the spectrum are the understandable reactions of people coming to terms with a serious disease. They respond with tears, frustration, bewilderment, anger and feelings of depression. Rachel recalls sitting on the floor weeping because she felt terribly ill in ways which no one could explain to her:

◆ Oh, I felt so awful. I remember one time my mum found me sitting crying and she said, 'Rachel, what's wrong?' and I said, 'I don't know.' I was just sitting there and the tears were pouring down because I didn't know what was wrong. Nothing was working.

All the people I talked to had spent days in tears – sometimes of pain, sometimes of loss, but perhaps most often of frustration with an illness which no one could understand, explain or treat. Many, both men and women, cried during their interviews when they remembered the hardest times. All of the young people wept as they recalled their worst moments and their harshest interactions with people who did not understand what they were going through. Most talked about feelings of despair and thoughts of suicide. But they were also courageous, inventive and sheer bloody-minded in the way they observed themselves, and found ways of preventing themselves from sliding down into clinical depression. The fittest went for walks, some talked to their dogs, some listened to music, some meditated. Others called friends to talk out their frustrations. If necessary, they talked to themselves until they managed to attain a more positive frame of mind. They often laughed at themselves, and laughed at their attempts to remain sane – OK, it's black humour, but all of them are still going, even the ones who show only small signs of improvement.

Sometimes with ME come emotional changes which go beyond the occasional tears of frustration and days of depression. Most people admitted to an emotional fragility unlike any emotional state they had experienced previously; it lasted for varying periods of time and it felt part and parcel of the illness rather than a reaction to it. They wept more easily than before, crying buckets at sad films or tragic news stories. They found it more difficult to control their emotions, describing their emotional equilibrium as a delicate balance which was easily disturbed. The more ill they were, the more their emotions spiralled out of control.

Sometimes the need to weep was reported as part of a general exhaustion and weakness. People wept and despaired when they were most flattened and defeated by their physical symptoms. As their physical strength improved, so did their emotional resilience. Or perhaps emotional fragility may be part of the illness itself – a symptom with a physical cause such as fluctuating hormone levels following a viral infection or during women's monthly cycles. This seems to be what Chloe is talking about – a cyclical ebb and flow of strong emotion – as she weeps through the bad days and then finds the strength to carry on:

◆ I've had quite a few low points. I mean, it comes and goes. Sometimes I find it very hard. I get very emotional and feel physically drained. Sometimes I find I'm quite depressed at times; you could say about once a month I'm quite low. And then I pick up. But the thing about ME is you can be in a great mood, laughing your head off, and the next minute you can be crying your heart out. It's very difficult.

Of course, not everyone with ME spends a lot of time feeling sorry for themselves – quite the opposite. Here is Chloe again, housebound for five years and trying to overcome her tendency to get tearful:

◆ Even now I'm quite an optimistic person. I really believe I will work again but there are times, low times, when you think: 'When is this ending?' That's the hard thing. But what I try to do is just laugh as much as I can and try to get through the good times, and then when you're sad I just kind of go with it and think: 'Well, I'm sad today, I'm going to have a good cry,' or whatever, and I usually feel a bit better once that's happened. I find I can snap out of it, probably because I'm a positive person.

Chloe, like all but three of the people in my sample, has no history of depression or mental illness. She describes herself as a 'bubbly, happy, out-going, sociable person' until she became ill. And, like others, even at her lowest ebb, she is not listless, withdrawn or without interest in life. She keeps trying. She keeps on searching for ways to carry on:

◆ When I'm really low and there's nobody here, there's no
back-up, nobody to talk to, I'll get one of my videos out and
I'll just put a funny video on and that makes me laugh and
that gets me out of my depression. I find that works for me.
Bit sad, isn't it!

In some cases ME produces disturbing mood swings and
changes in the way people habitually feel and behave. It is interesting that given the myth about women with ME being
neurotic and hysterical rather than ill, those in my sample
who talked with the most obvious angst about the loss of
emotional stability and control were men, such as Alistair:

◆ My children were about 14, 12 and 8. There is one child
particularly that I was very close to. It was the first time in
my life that I lost my temper with him, to both our horror.
Because there were times I felt I was on a very short fuse,
I think they just got to know that dad wasn't well. They
maybe didn't know why, but they knew there were days
when my wife maybe said, 'Look, dad's having a bad spell
just now. Leave him alone.'

Liam, like Alistair, explains his extreme mood swings from
elation to rage partly in terms of unbearable long-term frustration with the limits imposed by his illness and partly as a
response to intolerable pain. His wife, Emily, agrees:

◆ I remember times of sheer frustration, and certainly cracking
up when his mood swings caught me at a bad time, when he
swung into a violent voice which was unlike him, a totally

different personality. But he tried to explain that the
headache which went with him was so fierce that he
wanted to lash out. He felt that his head was on fire
inside, burning.

Liam dismisses simplistic psychological or psychiatric explanations for his mood swings, proposing instead one
which admits physical damage and organic change:

I suppose the same way my memory was affected, there
must have been something that was damaged. That the
emotional part of one's mind could be affected – why not?

This intrusive state of panic, anger or overblown emotion
presents people with ME with two possible routes – either
they can blame themselves, turn inwards and become depressed, or they can act out their violent moods on those
around them. The agony of ME pushed Liam to express his
rage rather than trying to contain it:

I would get rid of it by exploding outwards more than letting
it seep inwards. The inward seeping is probably worse for
the individual. The outward explosion is worse for the
people around you.

In his interview he describes a car journey with his wife and
daughter in which rage explodes as the pain in his head
becomes unbearable:

◆ We were on holiday in the north-west and we were just
driving round and I could feel the pain beginning to come.
We got lost, and all of a sudden I couldn't handle this. It was
tension. I thought it was their fault and I couldn't continue
to drive. I said, 'Get out!' to my wife – like that. All I meant
was to change over but she got out and walked down the
road and I thought: 'Goodness, what's happened?' My tone
of voice was so aggressive and so unreasonable that she
walked half a mile down to the beach to get away from me.

Despair

Despair is present in every one of the transcripts. Everyone
reports feelings of hopelessness which at times overwhelm
them. Some manage to shrug them off, like Fiona who goes
off to do voluntary work when depression presses in on her.
But others, like May, often do lose heart:

◆ At the time it was like being shut in a box, feeling totally
trapped and you just couldn't see any way out. I just felt …
I wasn't exactly suicidal … but I couldn't see any point in
life. Yes, I had feelings of despair most of the time: 'What
on Earth is going on? Why does life bother to continue to
go on? I don't care if I wake up tomorrow or not.'

With despair comes the contemplation of suicide. Roughly
half of the people in this study had thought about killing
themselves at some stage. Although such thoughts were
usually fleeting and quickly dismissed, sometimes death
seemed preferable to persevering with an empty, pointless

life filled with an unexplained disability and the prognosis of an uncertain future. Jamie admits to phoning his GP one Christmas because he was so depressed that he feared he might try to end his life. Chloe breaks down when she talks about the despair which once or twice made her think about committing suicide:

◆ At my lowest – I'm getting upset talking about it – but at my lowest I did feel suicidal because you've lost your life, nobody understands you, the doctors aren't there for you and you just feel that nobody is there for you and that's the difficulty I find.

You feel nobody is on your side ... once I was so bad that I had to phone the Samaritans up and it's hard even talking about that because you think: 'Phoning the Samaritans!', but that's how really bad it became. I was just crying. I just didn't know what to do with myself and nobody was here. I don't know what started it all. I just thought: 'I can't take any more.' So I phoned the Samaritans. The woman was good; she really calmed me down. That really was the bottom. It was a horrible horrible horrible time. My husband doesn't even know I phoned the Samaritans. I don't want people to know how bad I got.

Chloe has had the support of an exceptional husband, 'fantastic' parents and a sister she feels close to. Despite this love and support, in part her transcript is a long cry of emptiness, loss and sorrow. She acknowledges how lucky she is, knowing others who carry on in a vacuum of loneliness, but she is aware that she does not have the emotional strength to go it alone:

◆ They've all helped me emotionally and physically with a lot
of things. I really don't think I could have done it without
them. If they weren't there, I'd be away. I'd have killed
myself, do you know what I mean? That's how bad it is.

Anecdotal evidence about the number of people with ME
who have committed suicide show that Chloe and Jamie
and the others are not alone in asking themselves whether it
is worth carrying on. Shepherd writes, 'Tragedies do occur,
with suicide being the most common cause of death. Such
suicides are clearly linked to the associated despair and
depression which may accompany ME/CFS.'[11]

This is ME, but who am I?

A few people talked about the impact of ME in terms which
go well beyond the emotional fragility described by Chloe or
even the uncontrollable rage and loss of emotional control
experienced by Liam and Alistair. As a survival strategy,
some felt it necessary to subdue their personalities and rein
in their previously exuberant selves until they hardly knew
themselves. They talked about ME destroying self-identity as
they observed their personalities metamorphose into something unknown and unrecognisable.

Jamie, a writer, illustrator and storyteller, talks about the
erosion of a vibrant personality which burnt too brightly
to be accommodated by the constraints of ME. Previously
creative and extrovert, he was a performer who was at home
on the stage, telling stories, entertaining children, working
his unique blend of drama, fantasy and humour. Over a

period of ten years of illness, he has turned inwards and become quieter and more reflective because he is not physically strong enough to be the person he once was. In his interview he spends a lot of time discussing the loss and the meaning of his public personality which once he regarded as a separate act, something apart from his self. Illness has brought an understanding that the 'act' is a fundamental and important part of himself:

◆ I regret the apparent passing of this person, this persona. I realised that it wasn't all an act. This was part of me.

Recently he has occasionally returned to the stage; a re-entry which has brought into sharp focus the need to accommodate two co-existing and conflicting personalities:

◆ I can gain access to the part of me that is free and creative and quite close to how children respond. So, yes, I can present that and I can access their imagination and in the end, sometimes, quite often actually now, we reach a sense of understanding. We're in the same place and we're on a wild journey of imagination which is terrific fun … One of the things I have to deal with which sounds irrational is that I can be more myself sometimes in a very public place, in a risky situation. I've got 30 or 60 kids in front of me. Sometimes it doesn't work but I know that not only can I cope but that I can reveal a lot more of myself. I can be myself using my imagination. But then I go home and shut it all down again.

Today Jamie lives with two personalities – the one who is a creative performer and who comes to life in front of an audience, and the quiet, inward-looking ME one who has to shut down his vivid imagination and retreat to a quiet, reflective, lonely place. It is only in retrospect, having tried to revive the performer in him, that he realises how much of himself he has lost through his illness. Recently, he has salvaged some of his true self but only while he is performing on stage, not in any other area of his life. There ME still dominates. When I asked him what was his greatest loss, he replied:

◆ I've lost a large part of who I was.

Only two people said that their self-identity was neither challenged nor diminished by the limitations imposed by ME. Alison is one of them:

◆ No, it hasn't changed my sense of who I am at all really because I don't define myself in terms of my activity. I mean, what I am isn't dependent on what I do. ME has taken huge amounts away from me but the thing is that's what my life is, that is what I'm given, and that is what I have to work with.

Ruth, another person with a strong spiritual life, says the same:

◆ I have learnt to give purpose and meaning to suffering, to detach myself from the losses and replace them with something else ... with love, joy and peace. These are my

new measuring sticks, not work, not skiing, not my former
friends, but self-empowerment, compassion and kindness.
You always have love, joy and peace no matter what shape
your body is in. Every time I have a loss, I let go of it and
come back to thinking: 'What other way can I feel joy?'
It's an anchor that's always there.

Each individual suffers different losses from ME. Each takes
something different from the experience. Everyone changes.
Some adapt – out of necessity. The lucky ones are like
shadows temporarily dislocated from the real people they
once were. They eventually snap back into place, managing
a near if not perfect fit. Others, perhaps the majority, reluctantly have to come to terms with a different kind of living.

CHAPTER **5**

An illness without a diagnosis

> The notion that a disease can be explained only by a
> variety of causes is precisely characteristic of thinking
> about diseases whose causation is *not* understood. And
> it is diseases thought to be multi-determined (that is,
> mysterious) that have the widest possibilities as metaphors
> for what is felt to be socially or morally wrong.
> SUSAN SONTAG[1]

At the time of writing, there is still no diagnostic test for ME.
The implication of this for patients and carers is central and
fundamental to our understanding of the experience of
the illness, and to the way people talk and write about it.
Since doctors feel that they cannot reliably differentiate
patients who have ME from those who have other illnesses,
including psychiatric ones, the best that can be hoped for is
a GP or consultant who is open-minded enough to listen
and believe, and who may offer a diagnosis of ME after elim-
inating other possible illnesses. But this experience is rare.
Most doctors are uncomfortable with an illness which they
cannot diagnose – some are wary, many are cynical, sceptical, dismissive and patronising. While there is some variation in the ways that doctors react to individuals who walk
into their surgery believing that they might have ME, for
the most part patients must brace themselves for the raised
eyebrow, the lack of eye contact, and the rapid opening of
the door to show them out. One doctor I know told me in

confidence that he and his colleagues sometimes write in such patients' notes 'WGROH' – 'We've got a right one here.'

Illnesses which are not yet understood are prone to attracting the wrong labels, especially psychological ones implying personal inadequacy and self-blame. Without a diagnosis there is no external validation of the reality of an illness or the experience of it. Accounts of severe symptoms may be perceived as inaccurate and exaggerated, or are twisted to become evidence of a psychiatric illness. And so, without an objective test result, people with ME can expect to have a hard time. When I asked Alistair, the GP who is also an ME sufferer, how many of his medical colleagues believed that ME was a real, organic illness, he replied, 'I think there's a fairly small percentage do.'

Alistair describes an illness without a diagnostic test as a doctor's nightmare. He is expansive about the difficulties he faces when a patient appears in his surgery wanting confirmation that he or she has ME:

◆ One of the problems at General Practice level is that a lot of my colleagues feel that if you diagnose someone as ME and they haven't got it, it's what we might call a 'hypochondriac's charter'. We certainly had one or two patients labelled with it – or they labelled themselves – and they were off for ages, and I ... some of them ... I'm very sceptical if they had it ... I think the worry is that because it's so vague and symptomless, a lot of people could talk themselves into having it because they see the advantage. It's a very dangerous diagnosis to make. It's a no-win situation really. You know, you've got this condition that can be totally disabling and yet it's not accepted. I think we'd all feel a lot better if we could say, 'Look, we've got a diagnosis to hand. We haven't got this uncertainty.' I think we'd all love it.

From his own experiences he reckons that he can recognise a patient with ME when he sees one:

◆ I think you get a kind of sixth sense and a feel, not only for the common symptoms but the way people describe their symptoms.

Some doctors, like Alistair, remain baffled by ME, but try to listen and help, but all the available anecdotal evidence suggests that they are a minority. The amount of scepticism which surrounds the illness is brought home by the fact that Alistair received little sympathy or understanding from his own colleagues at the practice. No one who has met Alistair could imagine him as one of life's shirkers. It is very relevant that he says:

◆ I had a lot of sympathy from my reception staff but not a lot of sympathy from my partners.

The road to diagnosis

Experience of acute and chronic illnesses encourages an expectation of a medical textbook model of diagnosis and treatment: people describe their symptoms and receive either an immediate diagnosis, or tests, results, sometimes further referrals and, finally, a label. With the label comes a description of the illness, a prognosis and, usually, treatment. Most important of all there is validation of experience. None of this happens with ME.

There are a number of understandable reasons why people continue to search for a diagnosis even after they suspect that the search is futile.

◆ Fear of the unknown is very powerful. The possibility of a serious, life-threatening illness causes anxiety and distress. People worry that something is being missed, or that they have an illness which can be treated. Out of the 25 people I interviewed, 18 spontaneously said that they wished they had cancer because then doctors would take them seriously and there would be hope of treatment.

◆ Knowledge is power. People want to be better informed. With ME, patients become the experts, often well ahead of their doctors in terms of knowledge and understanding. The isolation imposed by ME lends itself to library work, surfing the net, but doctors are either not interested, or do not have the time to keep track of the latest research developments.

◆ A diagnosis brings some degree of control even while knowing that the diagnosis is tentative and that there is no treatment.

◆ A diagnosis opens the way for contact with others in the same boat. Communication between people with ME is often a lifeline.

◆ Wrong labels are hurtful and misleading. The outcome of a wrong label can be a fruitless and distressing trek through

specialist consulting rooms, usually of the psychiatric variety.
Individuals end up with negative test results, no treatment,
and a fat file which labels them a hypochondriac or a shirker.

Everyone I talked to said that a diagnosis of ME, even if that
diagnosis was inconclusive, was better than no diagnosis at
all. As Jamie says:

◆ **It was very important to me that my doctor recognised that
I had ME.**

Many of the men, women and young people in my sample
went to extraordinary lengths and put themselves under
intolerable stress in their search for a diagnosis, or at least
a confirmation of what they thought was wrong with them.
But the path to a diagnosis, or at least to a nod in the direction of a diagnosis of ME, is not the same for everyone.
Around half of the people who took part in this study were
eventually given an initial diagnosis by an alternative practitioner or by a GP who was working privately using complementary therapies. One was given a diagnosis by a
psychiatrist (who would not use the term ME); nine diagnosed themselves after reading up on the subject and
making contact with others – a diagnosis which was eventually confirmed by a private GP or an alternative practitioner
(in one case after eight years); five were given a diagnosis by
a NHS hospital consultant, though none used the term ME,
preferring the labels Chronic Fatigue Syndrome or Post Viral
Fatigue; five were diagnosed by their GP; one had a sister
who was a nurse who suggested ME.

The ease or difficulty with which they managed to obtain a diagnosis seemed to be determined by two factors:

◆ the patient's gender, age and status in society;
◆ whether the doctor had any previous professional and personal experience of ME.

The most sympathetic doctors were those with friends or other respected patients with the illness. Two people described their own doctors in glowing terms. One of these doctors had had ME himself, and the other had a relative with the illness. Personal experience seems to make a significant difference to doctors' attitudes, but experience alone does not necessarily open the doors to a diagnosis or to support.

The role of gender and status

The ease with which people achieved a diagnosis depended on their gender, age, status and confidence. Their experiences with GPs and consultants ranged from a quick confirmation to rudeness, scepticism and disbelief.

In general, the route to a satisfactory diagnosis was not so traumatic or demoralising for the men as for the women and young people. With a couple of exceptions, for them the process was less like a game of roulette with an outcome determined by chance. For a few – those with a certain status in society – the process was swift and relatively painless. For others, it was fraught and prolonged with no satisfactory outcome. It is interesting that even the most confident men, who obtained a diagnosis easily, talk about the process of diagnosis as difficult and inextricably linked with the fear of being thought a malingerer or hypochondriac. Alistair worked out for himself that he was probably suffering from ME. His purpose in going to see the consultant in the Infectious Diseases Unit in Edinburgh was confirmation, and he went armed with a letter from one of the partners in the practice supporting his hypothesis. Alistair had no problems with this notorious consultant:

◆ I went to see Dr W just to say, 'Is this what I think it is?' He said, 'Yes.'

When I asked Alistair if he thought he was believed, he replied:

◆ Yeah, possibly because I told him right from the start that this is what I thought it was. I suppose he didn't get a chance to say it was all in the mind because I gave him a fairly long catalogue of symptoms and more or less looked at him and said, 'Don't you dare bloody tell me it's all in the mind or I'll belt you one.'

This is confidence speaking. Alistair is already one of the brotherhood. How many of us ordinary mortals can face a consultant in this way? However, even Alistair was given no further help. Dr W wrote one polite letter saying there was nothing more he could do. He was not going to see Alistair again.

Liam tells a similar story, although in his case he and the consultant (not the same one Alistair saw) began a dialogue

of a different brotherhood – that of academics – and discussed different causal hypotheses, later exchanging articles
as if they were in a seminar rather than a consulting room.
Again, rank and status play their part in the kind of dialogue which ensued:

◆ Because I was a professor they wouldn't think I was
   malingering because there wasn't any point … as soon as
   they saw I'm a professor they didn't try the 'I'm a doctor'
   routine and they knew I was going to shoot them down
   with logic.

When I asked if he picked up any hint of scepticism about a
real illness, he said:

◆ Not at all. Not in the least. They would have been dead.

Both Liam and Alistair entered the consulting room ready to
do battle if necessary and were confident of victory. Mike was
equally fortunate. He saw two GPs, both of whom were sympathetic. One would not use the ME label, but accepted that
Mike had a long-term post-viral problem. The other GP, with
personal experience of ME, was very understanding:

◆ You can go in and tell him the symptoms much as we're
   discussing now and he'll understand exactly what you mean.

This is not the case for others. The men without the status of
Liam and Alistair tell a different story. Fraser was not sent to
the Infectious Diseases Unit but to 'a clinic full of old folk'

where he was put on a treadmill and given blood tests. It took weeks and weeks for the results to come back – all negative. So began the typical round of consulting rooms with no doctor willing to give him a diagnosis.

◆ I was getting nowhere, you know. No one would say to me, 'Mr C, it appears you've got ME.' They kept coming up with the line, 'There is no clinical diagnosis for ME', so they wouldn't tell me that's what it was. Just 'a sort of viral thing'.

I asked Fraser if any doctor ever used the word ME. He said not.

Jamie, like Fraser, entered into a protracted process of debate and discussion with his GP before a diagnosis was finally agreed. He had read up on the subject, knew how often it was dismissed and trivialised, and said how much it mattered that his GP labelled his condition as ME. But the GP was not interested.

◆ When I couldn't tell him what I thought, or what I thought of how he was treating me, I would write to him. He didn't respond directly, but he'd answer me the next time I saw him.

He told his GP about the impact of each consultation and how he felt he was misunderstood until, over a period of years, the relationship finally became more positive:

◆ I have sometimes put a lot of weight on him, or taken his time. I mean, I have been suicidal more than one time. One

Christmas was particularly bad and he phoned me on
Christmas Eve to see how I was.

Diagnosis is thus linked to understanding and to validation.
As Jamie says:

I just needed someone who knew how bad I felt.

The women in my sample had more varied experiences,
often with apparently random outcomes. Some obtained a
diagnosis fairly quickly. Some had to engage in a protracted
dialogue as they tried to persuade their doctors to believe
them and to take their illness seriously. Others did the soul-
destroying round of consulting rooms and were offered
psychiatric labels and antidepressants. For them the most
important factor was the personal experience of the GP or
consultant. Lizzie, whose GP was the same as Mike's,
describes her doctor as 'kind and wonderful'. Alison says
her GP readily offered a diagnosis of PVFS, never ME, but in
general was supportive.

On the other hand, Janet reports a long, fruitless and
demoralising debate in which her doctors were:

Apathetic and baffled. None of them could give me any
inkling as to why I was so poorly. I think they switched off.
Hopeless really.

Even her GP husband was hostile and offered neither
support nor understanding. Finally Janet accepted responsibility for her illness and, rather than fighting her way

79

round the consulting rooms, chose her own alternative road to recovery. She is not bitter about the experience, but is one of several people who describe ME as a turning point in their lives. In contrast, Denise desperately wanted a diagnosis. She was lonely, frightened and leaned heavily on a GP who finally blacklisted her out of exasperation. Like others, she then began on the lengthy round of referrals to private doctors, psychiatrists and alternative practitioners in her attempt to get a diagnosis and help. Finally, she found a chiropractor who agreed that she probably had ME. Denise remains bewildered by the difficulties she encountered:

◆ I thought that doctors were there to help us. You know, you're led to believe that that's what they are there for.

The GP's perspective

Alistair is interesting on the subject of gaining a diagnosis. On the one hand, he admits how tough it is for people with ME to walk away from a consulting room without a diagnosis:

◆ People are unable to work and they probably get [medical] certificates saying debility or depression or something. I mean it's a tremendous blow to that person's ego when they are off with something that no one is believing them.

But he also acknowledges that in the surgery, as in consulting rooms, character judgement enters into the equation. This comment is relevant to anyone who expects the process of diagnosis to be fair, consistent and rational because in fact the validity of our symptoms are weighed against our previous medical history and the doctor's personal opinion of us as people:

◆ It's often a matter of knowing your patients. I think you're always influenced by prior knowledge. If I saw someone who I knew, normally a bloke – and even women too – who was rarely at the surgery, you know that something is obviously wrong. Maybe they attend once every two years with sinusitis or something like that. When these people start coming with something that is so vague, then you say, 'Oh, there's got to be something here.' But if you've got a frequent attender, and we all have frequent attenders, then I think it's much easier to say, 'Oh, it's down to stress, anxiety and the fact that they're just not managing.' Yeah, I think that's right. I think that's one of the big problems which will always be faced by ME sufferers. Whether these people get it more easily than the copers, I don't know.

In effect, Alistair is saying that previously fit, macho men who rarely bother their doctors are going to be given a diagnosis of ME more readily than a woman who has had previous health problems. This comment from Alistair is consistent with what the people in this study report. A diagnosis is dependent on gender, age and status as well as individual doctors' judgements of us as people.

Diagnosis for young people

Compared with men and women, children and young people have the hardest time of all as they search for someone who accepts that they are ill, acknowledges the severity of their suffering, and understands the impoverishment of their lives. That young people have a much harder time obtaining a diagnosis of ME than adults is a reflection of their status in society. Also, there are still many doctors who do not accept that young people can suffer from ME. The clear message which emerges from the interviews is that nobody believes that these young people are genuinely ill. They are referred to psychiatrists, not ME specialists. They are forced through graded exercise and cognitive behavioural programmes. They are told that they have school phobia, anorexia, or that their mothers are keeping them ill by being overprotective.

It took Chris eight years to get a diagnosis; Jessie initially diagnosed herself; Kirsty was diagnosed eventually by a private practitioner; Josh was variously diagnosed by his GP as school phobic or anorexic. Rachel (whose appalling story is told in detail later) was diagnosed by a GP with ME.

CHAPTER 6

Not real or acceptable

Nothing is more punitive than to give a disease a meaning
– that meaning being invariably a moralistic one. Any
important disease whose causality is murky, and for which
treatment is ineffectual, tends to be awash in significance.
SUSAN SONTAG[1]

Most people with ME sometimes wonder if they have a real
illness. Cartesian theory, in which the body and mind are
considered separate, still has a profound impact on the way
doctors are trained today, and on the way society thinks
about illness. 'Real' illnesses are physical, organic, visible and
obvious whereas illnesses that have variable symptoms or
that cannot be conveniently labelled are doubted and dis-
credited. A plaster cast or a rash make a condition real – and
acceptable. Doctors remain uncomfortable with symptoms
that cannot, in their terms, be objectively verified with a test.
Which leaves people with ME in quite a mess.

Every single one of the interviewees talks about the problems of suffering from an illness which is without obvious
signs of disability which others could perhaps understand
and relate to. Only the tone varies, from tolerant acceptance
through fuming rage to tearful despair. How can you be
disabled when there is often no measurable outward sign of
disability? As Fiona says:

> If you see somebody with a broken leg then you know that's the cause and there's a time limit. But with something like ME, you don't really see anything physical apart from you know they're not right and they're tired.

Even Fraser, who quickly gives up trying to explain himself, admits how hard it is when comments about his illness are wide of the mark:

> People would say, 'I hear you're not feeling great.' To them I would look just as I did a year before. I'd look fine standing up and looking at them and talking to them. I would try and tell them, 'Well, it's sort of like this,' and they're sort of, 'Oh, it's that ... what do you call it? ... I read about it in the paper.' That sort of thing. But it really meant nothing to them unless you had an arm hanging off or a broken leg or six stitches. They wouldn't know.

An organic illness

There is mounting research evidence that ME sufferers do have physical abnormalities. Though the *cause* of the illness remains elusive, numerous biological abnormalities have been reported in:

♦ Immune function – in the form of cytokine overproduction or poor cellular function;[2]
♦ Brain and CNS – with possible involvement of the basal ganglia,[3] or the functioning of the blood-brain barrier;[4]

- Muscle – in the form of oxidation defects,[5] or post-exertional deficits;[6]
- Autonomic functioning – as neurally-mediated hypotension;[7]
- Hormonal function – most prominently at the hypothalamic-pituitary-adrenal axis;[8]
- Neurotransmitter function – particularly sensitivity to acetylcholine;[9]
- Neuropsychological functioning – including impaired working memory and information processing unrelated to psychiatric illness.[10]

Despite this evidence of biological abnormalities, and the acceptance of the reality of the problem at the highest clinical and academic levels, medical opinion on the ground is slow to assimilate it, preferring to cling to the myth of ME as primarily a psychological disease. The ME patient is in a precarious position when it comes to acceptance. While most people in the UK have now heard of the illness, and many know someone who has it, it does not yet have the same status as conditions such as heart disease or rheumatoid arthritis. Speaking at a recent American College of Rheumatology Annual Scientific Meeting, Dr Frederick Wolfe dismissed both ME and the related illness fibromyalgia as 'the end of a spectrum of symptoms ... of what appears to be distress.' Interestingly, he went on to say that ME exists only because our present society 'allows' it to exist. 'Historically, past societies have allowed other conditions. In the latter part of the nineteenth century, people had something called "hysterical paralysis" – they had fits. They don't have it any more because it's not a legitimate symptom or one that society allows.'[11] There are two main problems with this view. First, the growing body of research evidence to the contrary indicates that it is only a matter of time before ME is shown to be a real, accepted illness as defined in Wolfe's own terms. More importantly, society does not 'allow' ME in the way he suggests past illnesses have been 'allowed'. If it did, sufferers would not still be battling to be believed and fending off psychiatric labels. Dr Wolfe dismisses ME as a fashionable peg on which to hang a psychological malaise. He says there is a significant history of 'earlier psychological distress' in anyone who develops fibromyalgia. Other studies show that this is simply not true.

AIDS offers a good example of the way public perception of a disease changes over time, and with the advance of understanding and treatment. Once labelled the 'gay plague' which some claimed was sent by God to punish perverts, it carried a stigma which in some ways is comparable with that attached to ME at the moment. However, with new medical understanding, and a hard-hitting campaign involving HIV-infected people and the gay community taking to the streets, its status and meaning slowly changed in the public consciousness. The media modified their messages and part, if not all, of society followed. But in terms of its meaning and status in society, ME is stuck where AIDS once was. It is the Cinderella of illnesses.

The language of ME

There are a number of different names for the illness that most interviewees call 'ME', and these are used fairly hap-hazardly in the literature. One variant is 'Post-Viral Fatigue Syndrome' used by some doctors who believe that it is a self-limiting fatigue state following a viral infection, al-though this does not describe the experience of most suf-ferers. Again, the name adopted by many in the medical profession is 'Chronic Fatigue Syndrome' because one, but only one, of its main symptoms is overwhelming exhaus-tion. In the USA it is called Chronic Fatigue and Immune Deficiency Disorder (CFIDS). There, many people receive a diagnosis of fibromyalgia – a diagnostic label used for patients with severe muscle pain where there is no obvious rheumatic or arthritic condition – if the dominant symptom is pain. It is not yet clear whether fibromyalgia and ME are different presentations of the same illness. In fact, it is prob-able that the term 'Chronic Fatigue Syndrome', used by most medical professionals especially in Britain, is an umbrella term for a cluster of related illnesses which have different causes, different symptoms and different prognoses. One of these illnesses is ME, characterised by long-lasting fatigue hours or days after exertion, pain and a clear cluster of other symptoms.

A central problem concerns the word 'fatigue' which doesn't come close to describing how sufferers can feel – comatose might be better. Those who are severely affected – and others on bad days – are so tired that they can barely keep their eyes open. It is stone-cold tired, feeling endlessly and relentlessly drained. It is ill-tired, a pervasive, deep-rooted, sick, horrible sort of tired. Like most people with ME, I have acquaintances who say, 'Oh, I feel tired at 4pm too, and would love a snooze.' But that's not it. People with ME are so finished that they *have* to lie down. There is no other option. Minds and bodies do not function. There is pain and malaise. Without a period of sleep or deep relaxation, the rest of the day is a total wipe-out. As Josh says, if he is forced to carry on functioning at times when his body is shouting 'Stop', he pours sweat and his body literally shakes in compensation for an effort which is not sustainable. This is nothing like fatigue.

Finally, negative messages about an illness and the people who have it are common until a disease becomes accepted and integrated into a culture.[12] Derogatory labelling is a powerful way of discrediting a disease before it is understood: HIV and AIDS were frequently written about as the Gay Plague, and recently I heard that Repetitive Strain Injury is called Limp Wrist Syndrome by some doctors. For ME, Yuppie Flu was a favourite with the media for a very long time, suggesting that it was a fashionable and trivial illness reported by the middle classes, especially women, who had nothing better to do than complain about a bit of stress and tiredness. The facts do not square with this description, yet the label stuck and is still used. Other labels are equally hurtful such as the description of ME as an illness suffered by 'four-star people with five-star ambitions'. The message implicit in all these labels is that people who are ill are somehow to blame. Recently, Showalter[13] has described ME as on a par with phenomena like recovered memory, alien abduction and satanic ritual abuse. This is an interpretation of ME, written by an 'expert', which makes pure conjecture appear more valid than genuine, personal accounts of illnesses.

My own GP was very fond of the word 'psychosomatic'. She would say, 'You do have a tendency to somatise your symptoms.' Because my son weighed eight stone when he was over six foot tall, she used the label 'anorexic', despite our telling her, repeatedly, that even with nausea he ate and ate and ate. Ruby, Kirsty, Josh, David and Rachel were all told that they were 'school phobic' at some point by a doctor – that's *all* the young people still at school whom I inter-viewed. Both Ruby and Kirsty talk about how much they loved school, but such protestations fell on deaf ears. The other common label thrown at young people, explicitly by their peers, and implicitly by teachers and doctors, is 'skiver'. Josh describes how when he could not concentrate in the classroom, he was told by teachers that he was stupid and was not making any effort. Staff accused him of inventing illness to avoid his work and his peers taunted him. Rachel's report of her teachers' comments sum up all the issues about language which have been discussed here:

◆ You're skiving, aren't you, Rachel? There's nothing wrong with you. Come on, I get tired as well, you know. You just don't want to do any work.

Marilyn told me that her son David was called a 'confidence trickster' by a church minister. She herself was labelled a 'neurotic mother'.

Not being believed

The need to be believed is critical for young people. Initially they cannot understand a world in which reason and rationality do not prevail. But their expectations of doctors, teachers and other professionals, once naïve and trusting, change during their search for someone who believes them to one of cynicism and despair. In her short interview, 14-year-old Ruby uses the phrase 'faking it' seven times. Doctors, teachers and peers all think that she is imagining symptoms or deliberately misleading them by pretending to be ill in order to avoid school. She says:

◆ I'd see these looks on their faces. Like they don't say, 'By the way, Ruby, you're faking it', but they just give you this look like, 'We're not interested, go home, and quit this game.' But I can't because it isn't a game. They said I was scared of going to school, but I like going to school.

When Ruby's symptoms intensified, she still wanted to be there:

◆ Even when I was being sick and when I had fits in school, I wanted to get up and go back to my class.

For all the young people the lack of a diagnostic test has disastrous consequences. The bottom line is that they, even more than adults, are not believed. One of the most commonly repeated themes in their transcripts is their incredulity that adults in the medical and educational professions refuse to believe them and respond appropriately when they tell them that they are too ill to attend school, too ill to cope with the cognitive demands of a limited timetable or home tuition, and too ill even to interact with their peers. These are neither the truants who are disenfranchised with the education system, nor the less serious absentees who may use headaches or stomach pains as an excuse to stay away occasionally from school or from subjects which they dislike. It is so easy to make the distinction between the two groups. Young people who are school phobic or who are skiving for a while, come back to life in the evenings and at weekends, showing normal energy levels and going out with friends. Young people with ME are more ill after school because of the energy expended in getting through the day. They are ill every weekend. They do not manage out of school activities or social engagements with friends. Instead they lie in bed trying to recharge their batteries so that they can get through some of the weekdays in the classroom and playground.

CHAPTER 7

The psychiatric fallacy

The power of the myth was dispelled only when proper
treatment was finally developed, with the discovery of
streptomycin in 1944 and the introduction of isoniazid
in 1952.

SUSAN SONTAG (on TB)[1]

The debate about the psychological versus organic origins
of ME rolls on, as it has since the 1980s, despite the growing
evidence of organic causes. Williams[2] cites 17 key papers,
many published in prestigious journals such as the *Lancet*,
which show how ME differs in objective, quantifiable ways
from depression and other psychiatric illnesses. There is no
evidence in any of these studies of the often cited maladaptive attitudes and behaviours, nor of a phobic avoidance of
activity. Far from being switched off and apathetic, people
with ME, unlike people who are depressed, do not lose interest in life; they are desperate to claim back lives they found
stimulating and satisfying. Inevitably though, as with any
other chronic illness, a proportion of people with ME do go
on to develop clinical depression. But this depression is secondary to ME and not its cause. The distinction is crucial,
yet many healthcare professionals continue to maintain that
symptoms are *caused* by psychological, psychiatric or personality problems.

Looking back in time, there are a number of well-
documented precedents for the classification of a disease as

a psychological disorder at the same stage in its medical understanding. We need to remember what it was like for patients with leprosy, tuberculosis, multiple sclerosis, rheumatoid arthritis and schizophrenia before their diseases were explained and treatments or palliatives were discovered. Susan Sontag writes cogently about the gulf between the reality of tuberculosis and the enduring myths and metaphors which distorted and romanticised the disease before it was understood.[3] The same is true for rheumatoid arthritis. Dr Russell,[4] speaking at a recent ACR (American College of Rheumatology) scientific meeting said that when he first became interested in fibromyalgia, he reviewed the literature on rheumatoid arthritis and found that during the 1920s and 1930s, before the disease had been shown to cause joint destruction, medical opinion suggested that it was a psychological disorder. A recent report on schizophrenia sends out many echoes of what is happening to ME patients today.[5] The 40-year fall-out from RD Laing's book *The Divided Self*,[6] in which he postulates that the cause of schizophrenia has its roots in relationships with others, especially within families, is the single simplified notion that 'families cause schizophrenia'. Marjorie Wallace of the schizophrenia society Sane, says, 'After all these years, we still hear of parents being asked by their GP if they argue a lot or when they last had sex – at a time when they're seeking help, trying to cope with the fact that their child has been diagnosed with schizophrenia. They have this double burden of suddenly finding that someone they love has become strange and hostile, and then they're told it's all their fault.' This is so familiar to those with ME (or fibromyalgia). Dr

Ernesto Vasquez, speaks of his own experience, 'If I am in a wheelchair, there is a ramp for me to go up. If I'm diabetic, I can request a special diet. Fibromyalgics don't quite belong yet.'[7] Like all the people I interviewed, he argues that when people with a 'mystery' illness continue to search for a cause for their illness, they are searching for validation and acceptance.

Medical debate and research is dominated by psychiatrists and psychologists, some high-profile, who repeat over and over again that ME has its origins in 'biopsychosocial' factors.[8, 9] Translated into lay language, this means 'all in the mind'. For instance, one critique of the influence of psychiatric models of ME suggests that they were highly influential in the much criticised 1996 Report of the Joint Royal Colleges on Chronic Fatigue Syndrome,[10] to the exclusion of other biologically-based medical viewpoints. The report cites 256 references to psychiatric papers, half of which were written by people closely associated with the working group. Despite concerns about the methodology used in these studies, as well as other flaws in the reported research, and despite the absence of reference to the growing body of evidence concerning the biological abnormalities underlying ME, the UK medical establishment, government departments and much of the media seem to be in thrall to a psychiatric interpretation of ME.[11] The outcome is that only a small number of controversial treatments are on offer, based on this model, which are dogmatically imposed, and which most patients reject because they are ineffective or harmful:

◆ Cognitive therapy to realign supposedly distorted 'core' views or delusions which ME sufferers hold about their apparently imagined ill health.

◆ Imposed graded exercise to correct deluded beliefs about the necessity of rest, pacing and monitoring to prevent a deterioration in symptoms.

◆ Antidepressants to cure psychological illnesses. (Since only 10–15 per cent of people diagnosed with ME may be suffering from depression,[12] for the remaining 85 per cent antidepressants may prove either useless or harmful.)

The psychiatrists and psychologists who dominate the ME scene in the UK seem to refuse to acknowledge the reality of the illness, and its impact on the quality of life of sufferers.[13,14] Williams concludes: 'If [they] continue to ignore what is now world-wide evidence, they will be universally seen to be unscientific; they will continue not "to see the world as it actually is", and the consequences will continue to be disastrous for those with ME/CFS. In the interests of science, if not of humanity, this can no longer be tolerated.'[15]

The fall-out from the psychiatric fallacy

One of the strongest messages to emerge from this study is that people with ME feel insulted and demoralised by the suggestion that their symptoms have a psychological origin and, in the wake of a diagnosis of a psychological disorder, they feel defeated and trapped by treatments which do more harm than good. Denise describes the symptoms she was coping with when she went to her doctor – intolerable stabbing pains in her head, light and noise intolerance, nausea, an inability to wind down, agitation, insomnia, numbness in her fingers and hands, and the usual prostrating exhaustion. Her GP sent her to a psychiatrist who prescribed a series of antidepressants, substituting one for another when each made her feel worse. She told him:

◆ I don't need things like that. I'm not depressed although I admit I do feel down because I don't feel well. Not the other way round.

Describing the cumulative effects of the drugs she says:

◆ I felt a total mess. I tried to go out to do the shopping but had to be brought back. I couldn't travel on the bus. I lost my confidence. I wasn't getting any sleep. If I wasn't feeling sick, I was being sick. I found myself shaking.

Finally, she went privately to a chiropractor who suggested she was suffering from ME and accompanied her to an ME meeting where she recognised her condition in the accounts of others.

The unanimous consensus from the stories here is that referrals to psychiatrists were of no help. Phil agreed to referrals to psychologists and psychiatrists only after a deepening of the depression which gripped him as he became more and more ill. None of them reflected back an accurate perception of his illness, nor did they offer support or any other help:

◆ As the years went by I became more and more irritated with this focus on my mental state, instead of what for me was clearly a physiological illness first and foremost, and it wasn't being treated in that way. They would say things like, 'Ah, but the antidepressant isn't just for your mood, it will also help you sleep at night' and this sort of stuff. I wasn't convinced but, yeah, I colluded to the extent of thinking: 'If it's this or nothing then I'll try this.' The one that had the most major impact was the old-fashioned tri-cyclic amitriptyline. The psychiatrist started me off on 10mg and eventually bumped it up to 200mg. He used to say things like, 'You might struggle to make out the number of the bus you're waiting for if you're taking this.' And I went back to him and said, 'I'm not struggling to make out the number of the bus, I'm struggling to make out the bus.'

One of the problems with being told repeatedly that you are suffering from depression, or some other psychological disorder, is that you begin to believe it yourself. In my sample, the majority of the women at some stage questioned whether or not they were genuinely ill. Even Fiona, a confident, professional woman, and one of the very few to be given a prompt diagnosis of ME, began to doubt its validity one year into the illness, saying that she had 'no physical symptoms' although, in fact, she was suffering from joint pains and 'great fatigue' which left her unable to plan anything in her life:

◆ I was off work for over a year. Because there wasn't a lot known about ME at the time, you felt you were justifying yourself continually. You had no physical symptoms to show for it apart from losing quite a lot of weight. Other people would say, 'Oh, you're looking well.' But you know you were putting on make-up. You kept the flag flying in that way. It was very difficult and I started to think: 'Well, is it me? Is it all psychological?' I began to think it must be me.

With the doubt comes self-blame

Fiona describes the 'psychological element' in the following way:

⬩ When you begin to suspect that you may really have a psychological disorder, this can make you feel you're an inadequate person; that there must be something weak about you to make you prey to this. Of course, there's going to be a psychological element because if you're off work and your life is disrupted, it would take an incredible person not to become psychologically affected because at times you think: 'Well, am I always going to be like this? What kind of life will I have?'

Eighteen-year-old Rachel says the same thing. After appalling treatment by the medical establishment over five years, she says:

⬩ I'm not denying I've got psychological problems, but I think it's not cause and effect. It's Dr T's view that I'm ill because blah blah blah blah. But when you turn around and say to them, 'If you were stuck in your bed how many hours, or you relied on your dad or your brothers or someone to put you places, don't you think you would feel just a teeny bit depressed sort of thing?' They get very defensive.

Like Fiona, Rachel was made to feel that having ME (and hers is one of the most severe cases I have encountered) was her fault:

◆ Because I haven't got better, because I'm not walking, it's psychological. Now that I'm a bit better, I'm getting angry.

When I asked her if she had the energy to be angry she said:

◆ I'm trying damn hard to find it because I'm sick of being treated like dog poo under their feet. Because I have an illness and it's just as much an illness as AIDS or leukaemia.

Despite the evidence which informs us that ME is different from depression and other psychiatric disorders in a number of recognisable ways, patients remain vulnerable to the suggestion that their disease is caused by an emotional state or by personality problems. Ironically, it is not only orthodox psychiatrists who promote an essentially psychiatric origin of the illness. Many alternative therapists also promote the view that an emotional predisposition has caused the disease, and, like lambs to the slaughter, people go to purge their 'bad' emotions and cure themselves by admitting that they 'need' to be ill. To link disease with personality is, in effect, to blame each person for their illness. Those who are fit judge those who are ill and find them lacking. This philosophy makes disease a punishment. 'Such preposterous and dangerous views manage to put the onus of the disease on the patient and not only weaken the patient's ability to understand the range of plausible medical treatment but also, implicitly, direct the patient away from such treatment.'[16]

When it is finally understood, the cause of ME may indeed be found to be in the mind, but not in the sense used by the psychiatrists that have caused so much grief. The earliest descriptions of ME and indeed some current evidence suggest that it may be caused by a disturbance or malfunctioning of the nervous system which may result in heightened pain perception, fatigue and emotional fluctuations consequent upon a physical illness. In other words, while the cause of our symptoms may be situated within the nervous system, those causes are due to physiological abnormalities not a psychiatric illness.

The less we understand a disease, the more it is likely to be classified as a psychological, mental or emotional illness. It is part of the cycle of medical understanding. 'Theories that diseases are caused by mental states and can be cured by will power are always an index of how much is not understood about the physical terrain of a disease.'[17] At the time of writing, the cause of ME is still being researched and debated, and sufferers continue to pay the price of that lack of knowledge.

PART 2

Dialogues with a disbelieving society

CHAPTER **8**

Who believes you?

> When I was in the throes of ME and trying to explain the
> symptoms, you could see the shutters coming down. They
> were not going to listen any more. I always wished that I
> could find some telling phrases that they could relate to
> and understand, but I think it is totally impossible for
> people who haven't had it to understand. Now, a broken
> leg – people can look at it and say, 'Oh, that'll be sore',
> and be sympathetic; childbirth – 'That will hurt.' But with
> ME there is nothing.
> FIONA

Those with ME spend their lives staring at blank walls.
There are the walls of their bedrooms and living rooms
where they spend so much of their lives, but there is also
the impenetrable wall of incomprehension when they try to
explain to others how they feel.

People with ME are in a cleft stick. Either they try to
explain their illness knowing that their words will fall like
the proverbial seeds on barren ground. Or they remain
silent. It's a no-win situation, as Alistair says:

◆ If it was a well-accepted illness then it would be a very
   kosher thing to say, 'I've got ME and I can't do this, that
   or the other' but in general it's not a thing that people
   understand.

As Phil says, in the end it's easier to save his energy than talk to people who are not interested or who patronise him with their 'knowledge' of ME:

◆ I stopped telling people. I just don't bother anymore. I feel it's a waste of my time and possibly a waste of theirs. I think it's a question of channelling one's emotions and energies. I don't think there's any point in arguing with some guy in a pub on a Friday night for six hours as to whether ME is real or not. But I think those six hours could be better spent maybe influencing a committee, a journalist or somebody powerful within the medical profession. I don't see the point in trying to educate Joe Public.

Janet says the same:

◆ I don't waste any emotion on it anymore. I think I've got to guard what I've got. My energies, my emotions are very precious to me. I don't get involved any more. I think: 'Well, if they want to think that way, fair enough. I'm not going to get boiled up about it because it takes away my energy so I don't do it.' You have to learn to protect yourself.

Some of the difficulties of interacting with a healthy society are unique to ME because of a lack of a diagnostic test, but there is a more general gulf which Susan Sontag describes as the 'separate worlds of the sick and the well.' As Dawn says, there is a line which divides those who have experienced *any* disabling, disruptive illness and those who have not; when she suffered a major stroke, on top of ME, she encountered the same lack of understanding despite the visible signs of a limp and slurred speech:

◆ **The biggest gulf is between the healthy and the unhealthy. People make a thousand assumptions about you which bear no relationship to human history. Everyone who is sick is isolated from mainstream culture.**

And beyond this divide there is another which separates people who have encountered *any* trauma, tragedy or suffering in their lives, and those who are blithely skating along its surface. The people in Ruth's spiritual community accept her because many of them have suffered too, albeit in different ways. Even though they do not understand fibromyalgia, they are not put off or frightened by her illness:

◆ **To be a friend in my life you need to have gone through a crisis or be going through a crisis … In some ways no one will ever know what it [fibromyalgia] is like. So I don't have any expectation of having any rapport.**

Ruth speaks without bitterness. These are the facts. This is her reality.

To avoid negative, painful interactions, people with ME play a game in which they protect the healthy, robust, and intolerant from their own painful reality. They try to pass for normal rather than upsetting people by saying or showing just how bad it is. They protect friends and strangers alike because of *their* difficulties with the illness predicament, and in case they balk at the lack of an explanation for ME, except the one sufferers offer them.

Ruth says that she, like other disabled and disfigured people, make healthy people very uncomfortable:

◆ I scare the hell out of people by having a chronic illness. It's like: 'The fact of you scares me.' People need me to be better so that they can feel better.

Like a mirror, people reflect back to you images and facets of the person you are. In terms of what others observe, individuals may appear very different after years of living with ME. Some can adapt as illness reflects back a different image of a friend, relative or acquaintance. But many flee from the changes, especially friends and relatives who have been out of contact for a long time and may find it impossible to understand and adapt to a reflection so altered that they do not recognise the person they once knew – just as it may be impossible for the person with ME to cope with them as they come bouncing back into changed and reduced lives. Jamie says throughout his interview that he is unsure whether he has changed permanently or whether he is the same person trapped inside a sick body.

CHAPTER 9

Consulting rooms

> My impression of ME specialists is I reckon they get
> together at the end of the day and have a damn good laugh
> at all the things they've heard because they're absolutely
> useless, totally useless. I asked one guy if he had heard of
> Ampligen and he said, 'No.' I brought information to the ME
> specialist, a big hardback book and showed him an article
> about the thyroid. I asked him if he had seen the book. He
> said, 'No.' Specialists, eh? I find them patronising. As soon
> as they see ME written in your file then I think: 'That's you.
> You're buggered.' They won't take anything you say
> seriously.
> CHRIS

The narratives in this book reveal that for most doctors ME
is a heart-sink illness. The most common complaint is that
doctors do not listen. The second is that they do not believe
what patients tell them. The conventional model of illness –
tests, diagnosis, treatment – does not apply and so patient
and doctor lock horns, as Rachel explains:

◆ I would come away from doctors being told there's nothing
  wrong with me, what I was going through was nothing. It was
  a figment of my imagination.

When my elder son was ill with ME, my GP said that his
pallor (a ghostly shade of green) was because he was kept
inside too much. Note the wording, 'kept inside', as if he were
my prisoner. As if I *could* keep him in against his will. 'Don't be

so protective. Encourage him to run about in the fresh air more,' was the advice. Fortunately, my 13-year-old saw through her ignorance and chose to recover in his own way, in his own time. When my younger son suffered a severe relapse five years ago, lost two and a half stone, developed chronic nausea, vomiting and pain whenever he ate, our GP suggested Prozac and 'six slices of bread a day'. And so for three years we played the 'Avoid the Doctor' game, familiar to many parents of children with ME, because our interactions were so humiliating and frustrating, and the help offered was always inappropriate. We wanted to be completely free of doctors, yet dared not bite the hand which, in theory, cared for us, in case we needed them in an emergency, or if new symptoms developed.

While living for six months in London we found a GP who listened and acknowledged our son's suffering and the severity of his weight loss. She prescribed an anti-nausea drug which allows him to eat with less nausea and pain. She made a difference to the quality of his life. Back in Edinburgh, we have the stalwart support of a GP who has described our son, in writing, for the various benefits agencies, as 'a very fragile young man seriously ill with ME.' Maybe even she does not know how much her validation of his condition means to us. I describe these contrasting examples of practice to reveal the lottery of support and treatment people with ME encounter when they turn up in consulting rooms.

The doctor's perspective

Alistair, the GP who has had ME himself, opens a window on the attitudes of his profession to diagnosing ME as he chews over a number of the problems he encounters as a doctor dealing with patients who believe they have ME.

First, he worries about making a false positive diagnosis, something he calls 'a hypochondriac's charter.' So how does he separate the ill from the shirkers? He admits that his decision boils down to his previous knowledge of the patient, his personal opinion of them, and his hunch about whether there is something seriously wrong or not. As he admits, his judgement can be biased:

◆ We meet so many people who are making a real meal of their symptoms, and I think a lot of us, if we've nothing physically wrong to find, get a bit sceptical about it. A lot of people talk themselves into having it because they see the advantage. It's a very dangerous diagnosis to make.

'Wimps' (Alistair's terminology) and tough guys, even if they present with the same catalogue of symptoms, may be given different diagnoses. Alistair is right in saying that people *do* jump on the ME bandwagon – something ME patients would agree with. It is equally plausible to say that it is hard to differentiate someone with ME and a skilful hypochondriac. As we have seen, ME is a hard illness to diagnose. On the other hand, Alistair is admitting that previously fit macho types who do not clutter his surgery are more likely to be given a diagnosis of ME than females, 'frequent attenders' and those with complex medical histories. This leaves some genuine ME sufferers in quite a mess.

Second, he expresses concern about missing a case of clinical depression. Of course, he must rule out psychological and psychiatric illnesses, but is he correct in saying that depression can be missed 'because the symptoms are very similar to a certain degree to ME'? Probably most doctors would agree with him, but while there is some overlap between the two conditions, there are also crucial differences.[1,2] In my sample there was little evidence of the classic signs of depression. Even those who were very ill and whose lives were extremely limited had not given up and far from withdrawing from life were desperate to get back into it.

Third, Alistair says ME is a heart-sink illness because it is time consuming, unrewarding and low status, with doctors ending up as social workers unable to make their patients better.

◆ One of the reasons ME is not a huge priority is that there's a lot of work and time lost to it compared to well-known conditions ... Many of us haven't got the time to get involved. It's a vicious circle really. It's a thankless condition. I can't think of any other condition that is as thankless.

Yet, as is the case in my own family, the support of a GP can make a significant difference to the quality of life both of someone with ME and their carers. Even if a cure is not available, doctors can offer practical and psychological support, and validation. They can also offer the right advice about management at the onset of ME – very few people in my group were given appropriate advice in the first weeks and months, and as a result pushed themselves into a more severe, chronic form of ME by doing all the wrong things.

These patients are the very ones who will consume huge amounts of time in the doctor's surgery.

Doctors like to make people better. It is their allotted role. And so, when faced with someone with an illness which they do not understand, they feel impotent, as Dr Daniel Claw explains: 'Our job is to help and we feel helpless in the face of these diseases. Some doctors push patients away by saying they can't help, or subliminally by telling them their problems are all in their head.'[3]

Alistair is more open and sympathetic than most doctors because he has had ME. But his remarks about his colleagues are hair-curling. While he admits his own fallibility in diagnosing ME this is not the case for other doctors who *know* it is not 'real'. While he is not personally swayed by the powerful dogma of the reigning psychiatrists, he admits others are:

♦ It could influence a lot of people who have never had it. Knowing a lot of my colleagues, that would set their minds in stone. You know – 'This is a psychological illness therefore we're not interested in it at all. Get on with your life, you silly person.' That's a very dangerous thing to say. I think it really is a very real physical entity, but it's very hard to get acceptance amongst doctors who are scientifically trained, and to be scientifically trained you have a set list of symptoms and signs, and you come to a diagnosis. I think it's a terribly difficult thing. If you're lecturing to a symposium of doctors, it's very hard to say that there's nothing clinical to show because that's what doctors want and that's what we were trained for.

In fact, while scientists are trained to deal with things they do not understand, the clinician is uncomfortable and frustrated by having to make decisions about patients while in a state of ignorance. Fourteen-year-old Ruby, cynical and enlightened after her disastrous encounters with doctors, makes the sophisticated point that doctors need to acknowledge their own ignorance, as the best undoubtedly do:

They don't want to learn anything. They think they know it all and they don't want to believe in anything else. They think they know best. They wouldn't listen to my mum even though she was the one who knew what was going on. They always come up with a quick diagnosis or something or other. They didn't believe anything that wasn't in the sort of books they read. They read this whole book and if anything wasn't in it, it was fake or it wasn't real. I don't think they're bad. I just think they should be less cynical and go and learn. They think they know everything. They should learn more and read more books about different diseases and things they don't believe in. They should kind of wonder why they don't believe.

The patient's perspective

Many of the doctors described in the narratives behaved in ways which were cynical, unkind, wrong, rude, intolerant and damaging. There is no way of knowing how representative they are. A few people found their doctors supportive or non-committal, but these were the minority and most of them were confident, professional, articulate people who brought to the consulting rooms a status and confidence which defused medical arrogance. Or, like Alistair, they already belonged to the club. Alistair and Liam enter consulting rooms on equal terms with their doctors, ready for dialogue and, if necessary, confrontation. Others have disaster scenarios to relate.

There is not space here to include all the horror stories of people being insulted, struck off doctors' lists, wrongly labelled and reduced to tears of anger and frustration but below are a couple of examples. The stories told by the young people, *all* of whom were abominably treated by a number of doctors, are told together later (*see* pages 120–34).

Denise became ill after a viral infection in September 1997. She battled on, thinking nothing much of it. For three months she went back to her GP and was prescribed paracetamol. When her symptoms worsened and her mother requested a home visit, the doctor refused. Denise's mother walked into the surgery to demand that the doctor come to her daughter's home:

◆ **The receptionist told her I should be taken to the Royal Edinburgh because there was something wrong with my head. Yes, the receptionist.**

By this time Denise was nauseous, vomiting, and bleeding from the gums and anal passage. She had tingling and numbness in her limbs and stabbing pains in her head so she kept going back to the surgery, and repeatedly asked for house visits, because she was 'very very scared'. As a result, she was blacklisted by all the doctors in the practice. Her GP refused to see her, and when she asked to see another doctor in the practice she was refused because she was not his patient. Even the nurse blocked her:

◆ I went one day and I saw the nurse. I was really desperate. I said, 'You have to do something. I really am feeling bad.' I got literally chased out of the surgery. Dr C came out of his room and was really horrible to me. I came away feeling dreadful. I thought: 'Nobody believes me.' I felt they thought I was making it all up.

Denise deteriorated. She developed severe panic attacks. She was almost permanently in the 'tired but wired' hyperstate which is familiar to many people with ME. Terrified, she had no idea what was happening to her. Finally, her GP agreed to a consultation, 'sneering all the way through it', and referred her to a psychiatrist who diagnosed depression and prescribed in succession Prozac, Seroxat, Co-didamol, paracetamol, Ibuprofen, Zimovane, and Dutonin. The drugs made her worse, but the psychiatrist's response to her adverse reactions was, 'I can't understand why these tablets should do this to you – you're shaking away. You're just depressed, that's all.'

Denise now wonders how much further down this path of insult and injury she would have travelled if she had not been given a diagnosis privately. Here is one of Alistair's 'frequent attenders', turning up again and again in the surgery, seeking help, breaking down, weeping with pain and fear – the classic nightmare patient. But then perhaps she did not have the confidence to explain herself calmly and clearly. But how many people who are this ill do?

While most of the men fare better than the women in their interactions with doctors, those who are very ill are treated in a similar way. Chris, like Denise, not only battled with psychiatrists about the validity of his symptoms, but found that the ME label meant that other potentially serious symptoms were overlooked:

◆ I went back to see the guy who had sent me to the psychiatrist. I just got in the door and sat down and he said, 'Oh, I see you're getting on fine now. Well, there's no need to see you again.' That was it. That was the last time I saw anyone for years and years. I did go back to him about my throat. My tonsils had opened up. I said my throat was sore all the time and I had all these aches and pains, and he said, 'Oh, you look perfectly healthy to me.' And I thought, 'Gosh, don't I know my own body?' I couldn't speak to him so I wrote a letter saying: 'Could you refer me to an ENT specialist?' This was after two years of having him look down my throat and not doing anything ... I saw the ENT guy and I got the tonsils out quite soon. I remember the doctor came round and said they were the most disgusting tonsils she had ever seen. They actually broke when she took them out. I thought: 'Bloody hell, that's my GP's fault.' I think they categorise you as an ME stress person so anything you say, they don't have to take it seriously.

Chris's experience shows how having ME can result in dangerous neglect. Nor was that the end of the chapter. He suffered a haemorrhage and was re-admitted to hospital with a secondary infection.

If there were an award for the most damaging, off-the-wall interaction with a doctor, there would be plenty of nominations from the people I interviewed.

This is Chris, trying to tell his GP how ill he feels:

Chris: I'm not well at all.
GP: Well, you can't be well all the time.
Chris: Look, when I used to swim, I used to do lots of lengths. Now I can't do any.
GP: Next time you feel like that, just do more.

The GP took a throat swab, but failed to send it off:

You know he was just doing the gesture. Of course, no result came back.

And this is Kirsty:

I remember going to the GP. It was a lady doctor. I had put on a lot of weight because I was bedridden. I went along, and in an attempt to be normal and trendy I put on a pair of jeans and a denim shirt. She said at the end of the consultation, 'You know, you've put on an awful lot of weight, dear.' That was the last time I ever wore jeans.

And this is Phil, very sick, very distressed:

I can remember one occasion when I went down to the surgery and just poured my heart out. I said I desperately need something, please help me – or whatever. For the full seven minutes I rambled. At the end of the conversation, or the monologue really, he picked up his pen and prescription pad and started to write. I was overjoyed. I thought: 'Wonderful!' I didn't know and I didn't care what the prescription was for, but here was my doctor writing me something that was going to assist me in some way with how I was feeling. Then he said, 'This is for the cold sore on your lip, Phil.' And I realised he had been looking at me intently and it was nothing to do with the words coming out of my mouth but the herpes on my lip. That was the sum total of his contribution.

There are kinder, more useful and humane ways of dealing with patients with ME, as Alison explains when she lists exactly what she appreciated about her doctor's behaviour:

◆ She offered a prompt diagnosis of 'post-viral fatigue syndrome';
◆ She prepared Alison slowly for the possibility of ME, taking time since the illness might have been a short, self-limiting post-viral condition;
◆ There was no pressure to put on 'the brave smile' in the surgery;
◆ When Alison refused antidepressants, saying she preferred to practise meditation, her GP accepted it;
◆ There was no suggestion that the illness was all in the mind. This GP had already seen and treated a lot of cases of ME in New Zealand, and so was predisposed to accept the illness as 'real'.

Throughout the transcripts, people echo this last point. Doctors who have seen clusters of ME patients or have worked in specialist clinics or have known friends or family with ME, or have had the illness themselves are much more likely to be affirmative, informative and helpful.

Role-playing in consulting rooms

Alison and others talk about the need to role-play 'the good patient'. Alistair has already admitted that doctors make character judgements, preferring the stoic to the tearful, so the games may be a necessary part of the process of obtaining a diagnosis and support. Convinced that doctors may not be rude to 'good patients', and may not pounce with inaccurate labels, people ask themselves: 'How can I make this doctor listen to me? What signs will he pick up that will damn me? How do I behave to avoid being labelled neurotic or hysterical or a hypochondriac? How do I make him see me as a reasonable, sensible and sick person? Should I be bright and brave? Or can I reveal my real feelings of fear and despair?' It is like children in school who supply the answers they think their teachers want, rather than voicing thoughts which might conflict with the teacher's expectations. As Chris says, these games probably make patients more nervous and more likely to say something which offends than if they entered the surgery without the preliminary stage rehearsals. Yet facing the doctor can be very threatening:

◆ There is so much I want to say, and I imagine them reacting in a certain way so I'm planning everything ahead. I feel that they're going to dismiss anything that I do say and I'm going to have to fight my corner. It's very stressful.

When Alison's partner also developed ME, then the games had to be played, even with an understanding GP with prior experience of the illness. They had to 'work on her' to convince her. Alison judged that it was counterproductive to put on the bright-and-breezy-in-the-face-of-illness act:

◆ I stopped being positive, I started being a bit gloomier, and she started believing me again. But I kept the brave smile so she wouldn't think I was giving up.

What hard work it is! What a lot of extra thought, concentration and effort it takes to monitor her behaviour so that she does not fall over the trip wires of an inappropriate or condemning diagnosis! Alison was seriously ill by this time, and yet she had to calculate and achieve the correct balance of stoicism and sadness to maximise her chances of receiving validation. What a lot of energy used up in second-guessing doctors' reactions instead of just being honest.

One reason for the lack of stoicism (and why should ill people be stoic anyway?) is that emotional liability is a part of ME. Patients weep more easily, feel agitated, and experience panic attacks. There may be feelings of fear and anxiety bottled up for ages because there is no one there to listen. Then as the surgery door opens, men and women break down. Don't doctors know that they see people in their most vulnerable moments and not as themselves?

CHAPTER **10**

Young people and doctors

> Basically, they let people down. They let so many lives be
> wasted. There is no research. I'm sick of being treated like
> dog poo, of being trodden under their feet, because I have
> an illness … but all I get is, 'You're skiving, Rachel. There's
> nothing wrong with you. Come on, I get tired as well, you
> know. You just don't want to do any work.'
> RACHEL

The stories told by the young people should stop us in our tracks. All of them give cause for concern. The reported power struggles between the young who have little status in society and the doctors who are regarded by many – sometimes including themselves – as God-like is a hopeless one, with a predetermined outcome. Every young person in this study has encountered negative and dismissive attitudes. Most received inappropriate or harmful treatment.

Fifteen years ago, the story of Euan Proctor, one of the first cases of a young person with ME, provoked outrage, argument and endless newspaper column inches of debate about the validity of his condition. He was made a ward of court, removed from his parents, and taunted and tortured by the nurses and doctors who told him there was nothing wrong with him. His experiences in hospital must have been agonising beyond imagination. At one point, he was tipped out of his wheelchair into a swimming pool while nurses shouted, 'Swim! There's nothing wrong with you!' What has changed for young people with ME in those fifteen years? Not much.

'You have school phobia'

All the young people talk about the false diagnosis of school phobia. Typically, it is with this label that Rachel's story begins. She talks about the impossibility of articulating her physical and cognitive disabilities with doctors who had made up their minds, against all the evidence, that the cause of her illness was school phobia:

◆ I was only 11, and 11-year-olds don't know what is happening to them at the best of times. I was being told all these things, and I didn't know what was wrong with me. I couldn't figure out what was happening to me because I was being told that I was afraid of school, yet why was I still wanting to go?

If school did finally become unbearable, it was nothing to do with phobia. What Rachel describes is an environment which is agonising and exhausting for someone who is very ill:

◆ I didn't like school because of what was happening to me. I couldn't cope with school. I couldn't process all the information. I didn't have friends. It was just too much.

If Rachel had been school phobic, she would have bounced back to normal health at the end of each term, but instead she describes a family holiday to Disneyland as a nightmare in which she was wheelchair-bound, exhausted from the heat and the noise, and unable to cope:

◆ I remember looking at photographs afterwards and asking Mum, 'Why didn't I smile?' It was the heat and going round. Pure exhaustion.

Her doctors judged otherwise. Rachel was placed in a locked environment for children with severe emotional and behavioural problems. Here she was 'not allowed to be ill'. Yet she *was* very ill while trying to cope with highly-disturbed children in accommodation with 'bars on the windows and reinforced glass' which she describes as 'one of the worst places I've ever been in.' After several months she was discharged, not because the placement was judged inappropriate, but because the nurse therapists decided there was nothing physically or emotionally wrong with her. She was told she was not ill.

The next move was to a different secondary school and, when again she could not cope, she was sent to a residential school for children with learning problems where she deteriorated further:

◆ I was 15. This was the worst I had been. I had gone down and down. I was getting really ill. I had lost me. I'd lost the spark that was me. I'd just given up. I got a kitten and it kept me alive because I had something to live for.

Her GP, who told Rachel that she did not believe in ME, referred her to one of the 'ME specialists' in Edinburgh. He admitted her to a ward for children with infectious diseases. There was still no diagnosis, despite the evidence that she was steadily deteriorating – so much so that she was put on a feeding tube:

◆ I lost control of my head, my sitting, my balance. I had no muscle power whatsoever. I was using a wheelchair. I weighed 7 stone 10 pounds and was 5 ft 11 in. I jerked – I don't mean twitches, I jerked with so much pain.

Then the children's ward was closed. Rachel had been in hospital for almost a year. Now 16, she was moved to the HIV and Drug Rehab ward:

◆ It was a lovely experience. Alex coming through my door searching for fags and methadone at 5.30 in the morning. Pamela, a drug addict, came in raped one morning and I was holding her and she was crying – I'm holding her and I'm one of the patients. I lived with so many things in that ward. People dying. The methadone. The drink.

When I interviewed Rachel, she was back home after thirteen months in hospital. Her views of the medical profession are harsh. She knows first hand their ignorance, their dismissal of ME as a psychiatric illness, their arrogance. The consultant was, she says:

◆ A big bullfrog full of hot air. If you burst him, there would be nothing left. He wants to pump you full of drugs: 'There, there, you good patient, you're better now, go home. We saved you.' But I haven't got better.

Although she was spared a whole year in a hospital environment, Kirsty too was admitted to an inappropriate ward after she was diagnosed as school phobic. She ended up in a geriatric ward full of senile patients. Like Rachel she had to cope with ME *and* the madness of her environment:

◆ It was just a nightmare. I was 15 and I think the next person to me in age was something like seventy years older than me. You know, they were all about 85. They were geriatric. I mean somebody with ME lying for a week in a bed in a room, it was very hard to deal with. Those ladies were wandering about and one of them thought I'd stolen her cigarettes and I didn't have the energy to get out of bed, let alone anything else, but she'd wander over and raid my locker.

The ward was not just distressing and difficult; it was potentially dangerous. Talking about the behaviour of the same confused patient, Kirsty describes how she was almost smothered:

◆ She had a pillow one night and almost suffocated me. It was just a terrible experience. It was really quite horrendous.

Katy (a young woman who contacted me while I was working on this book) was admitted to a psychiatric hospital after she attempted suicide in despair at the severity of her symptoms which had kept her bedbound for three years. The fire alarm went off. A nurse herded her from her bed and tried to make her climb up a flight of stairs – she collapsed. But why *up* the stairs instead of *down* in the event of fire? Because setting off the fire alarm is an old trick to separate those with a 'real' illness from those who are laying it on with a trowel.

At the age of 14, exasperated and disillusioned, Ruby describes with venom the closed-minded attitude of the medical profession to children with ME. In her interview Ruby talks a lot about doctors not listening. She also makes the point that if a doctor cannot find evidence of any known disease, *and* fails to believe what the child is saying, it is reasonable that he should question the reasons for his own disbelief:

◆ They should kind of wonder why they don't believe it. And they should listen. It's as if they don't want to listen when they come and see you. If we're going through it, and they don't listen to us, they don't know what's going on. They just come up with something, 'Oh she's crazy,' things like that. I felt hurt.

In the end, Ruby gave up talking to doctors:

◆ I tried to explain to the doctors and then I thought: 'Well, there's no point, they'll label me this and that.' Everything I said, they'd use against me, like if I said, 'I feel sick,' and things like that, they'd say, 'Well, you're bound to say that because you want to stay off school.'

When I asked Ruby how she felt about doctors, two years down the line, she replied, 'I think they should all be sacked and burnt. Burn the doctors' books and write new ones with new theories in them.'

These stories show that doctors continue to individualise the experiences of young people with ME, instead of recognising common patterns, symptoms and suffering. Each young patient is pathologised in terms of personality defects and inadequacies, and described with psychiatric labels.

'It's all your mother's fault'

All seven of the young people interviewed were diagnosed as having a psychiatric illness yet all seven were eventually given a diagnosis of ME or CFS. As a result of medical prejudice and ignorance, parents are left to play a precarious game of keeping their children out of the clutches of doctors – particularly the psychiatrists.

Six of the young people I interviewed were living at home because they were too ill to take care of themselves. Of these six, five said their mothers had been accused of contributing to, or causing, their illness. At the mild end of the continuum are comments about mothers being over-protective, overcautious or neurotic. At the sharp end lies the diagnosis of Munchhausen's syndrome by proxy.

Mothers of young people with ME are in a difficult situation. Inevitably, as peer group support and friendship falls away, they become many things to their sick child – even if that child is in his or her teens or twenties. Mothers are the carers, cooks, cleaners and companions. They provide physical support, mental stimulation, moral support and social interaction. While it is inappropriate for mothers to intrude

too much into the lives of nearly grown-up offspring, sometimes there is no other option.

The closeness and intimacy which develops between
mother and child is as inevitable with ME as no doubt it is
with other chronic illnesses. Yet doctors see the mother–
child relationship as pathological rather than regarding it as
an inevitable outcome of the situation. The relationship is
viewed as warped and wrong. Mothers are both blamed for
their children's illness *and* become involved in a draining, demoralising battle fending off wrong labels, wrong diagnoses
and wrong treatments. Mothers do their best in a heart-
breaking situation, keeping their own emotions under wraps
as much as they can while protecting their children.

Protecting children from doctors

Marilyn lived under the constant threat of a medical intervention for her son which she believed would be harmful.
She stood up to the doctors, protecting David from their in-
terference. She describes her life as being under siege from
the medical profession – a state of warfare which lasted
many years. While she battled, she knew doctors and teachers all thought that she was at the root of David's illness; the
reason why he did not get better:

◆ I battled for two years with the education authorities, the
people who oversee children who are not going to school.
We had one doctor who was wanting to arrange family
meetings, blaming mum, implying it was a problem in-house.
I just wouldn't let her come to the door any more. I lived

under the threat of David being taken into care. I refused
point blank. We got a letter saying he had an appointment
for an hour and a half at this clinic and I knew that if they
were offering an hour and a half appointment, they didn't
know anything about ME. I flatly refused. I battled until he
reached the age of 16.

Throughout these years, David was profoundly ill, bedbound for two years, and unable to look after himself. His
life was a cipher, filled with pain, nausea and insomnia,
where even the sound of his mother's footsteps were intolerable. Marilyn says that despite this, doctors wanted to take
him away from his quiet home and put him in a bright,
harsh, noisy institutional environment over which he would
have no control:

◆ I knew it was inappropriate. I knew David was very
physically ill. It was nothing whatsoever to do with the home
environment, nothing whatsoever to do with mum. He was
very very physically ill.

The result of her stand against the doctors was that she was
labelled 'neurotic' and effectively blacklisted by the medical
establishment. She says of the other mums she knows in the
same boat:

◆ Most of them get up and fight on their [children's] behalf.

Ruby's mother, Ann, now with a diagnosis of Munchhausen's
syndrome by proxy, lives under the threat of her daughter

being taken into care. During her interview she broke down and wept as she talked about this wrong diagnosis:

◇ It's indescribable. I mean it is utterly indescribable.
All I can describe it as is mental torture. You know, there
you are with your sick child, and you're treated like a
total pariah. I mean, all these aggressive, hostile people
who should be helping you but in fact are doing the
absolute opposite.

Like others, she is incredulous and indignant at the ignorance and arrogance of the doctors with whom she came in
contact:

◇ ME is classified as a psychiatric illness so they approach
it with blinkers. This is their belief system. How could a
consultant paediatrician fail to see what are obviously
neurological symptoms? They are so brainwashed they
can only believe it's psychiatric.

Ann described how Ruby's condition had deteriorated over
six months to the point where she was bedbound, fainting
and vomiting. She confesses that she broke down in her GP's
consulting room, begging for a diagnosis. She was sent, letter
in hand, to the emergency department of the local hospital:

◇ We went along and I naively thought we were going to be
helped. I mean there have been so many points I thought I
was at breaking point, yet looking back I realise they were
only the tip of the iceberg. If I'd known what was coming,

you know I honestly think I would have shot myself because the horrors were unimaginable.

The horrors to come were hostility and an atmosphere of accusation on the ward from nurses and doctors. After several days, Ann was summoned by the doctor who said, 'It's a very serious case. It's imperative she sees a consultant psychiatrist.' Ann refused permission, Ruby remained on the ward, and Ann continued to be treated 'like a pariah'. Then one day she picked up the case notes which had been left at the end of the bed:

◆ I read it from cover to cover and I was horrified because of the total manipulation of evidence. They had omitted all physical symptoms and written it up as a psychiatric illness. It was a no-win situation. There were all these references to me. Whatever I did was distorted and things that were perfectly innocuous were given a twist. Things like 'Mother very attentive today.' 'Mother drew curtains round bed.' 'Mother didn't want child to take part in play activities on the ward.'

Ann suspected what was going on, gained access to Ruby's medical records, and there was the accusation in writing:

◆ There was a secret report about me. They wrote this totally fictitious damning report making out that I have Munchhausen's syndrome by proxy ... It has had a terrible effect because it destroys your life. It destroys the whole family's life. Because I'm on my own, it's even worse. If I had one other person who could help, but I was stuck in the house on my own because she was too ill to go out. I had to take medical retirement from work. She was ill all the time. She was up all night; I was up all night. I was exhausted all the time. This is the reality. It's so horrific. You do lose your marbles. It caused me to become depressed and it was the direct result of the report accusing me of Munchhausen's syndrome by proxy. So I am struggling with depression too and it makes me so very angry. It's an abuse of human rights. Others are going through the same misery as well. It is medical abuse. There is no other term for it. It is abuse by doctors of families. It is destroying.

Ann is now becoming ill herself. Like other mothers she is under the double strain of witnessing her child's suffering while fending off hostility from the professionals from whom she expected support. Ann's story is neither exceptional nor rare. Mothers of children with ME are still depicted as neurotic and overprotective, nor is it uncommon for them to be accused, like her, of Munchhausen's syndrome by proxy.[1,2] And Ann's agony has been picked up by Ruby who has followed the pattern of events. The 14-year-old now copes, not only with her own illness, but with her awareness of her mother's distress:

◆ Dr G wrote this whole horrible report about my mum. She didn't even know me. She hadn't even come to see me and she didn't know what I was like. It was just stupid because she didn't even know me. My mum got upset, got really upset about it, and she's still angry with the doctors.

Josh's father, Nelson, has much in common with mothers like Ann and Marilyn who talk about the problems of convincing doctors who do not believe them. This leaves him feeling vulnerable and responsible in case the conclusions he draws from his daily observations and interactions are wrong:

◆ At one point, our GP proposed that Josh might have anorexia. He was six foot two and weighed just over eight stone. It was not an implausible suggestion and certainly one that had to be ruled out. Of course, my reaction was: 'That's absurd.' He had great difficulty eating being both hungry and nauseous, but that is not a normal anorexic combination. I knew that Josh's only interest in food was how to eat it so that he could put on some weight and get his life back. He was ashamed of being thin. He wasn't anorexic. But I also knew that other loving parents had made the same mistake. Fortunately, our GP was prepared to come and watch Josh eat a large meal, and to observe that a combination of squeaky floorboards and an eccentric plumbing system would have made vomiting a highly public performance.

When anorexia was ruled out, depression was proposed instead. But Josh did not have the classic symptoms of depression. He had agreed to try antidepressants but reacted badly to them. Once again, Josh's father locked horns with the GP:

◆ In the end it came to a face off with the GP who wanted to
refer him to a consultant psychiatrist. Fortunately, we had
been in the ME process long enough to know that this
particular psychiatrist, and his department, denied that ME
existed and had a horrendous record of treating ME cases.
I refused to have Josh referred. It was the single most
important decision I made throughout his whole illness.

It was the right decision – but to take up a stance against
the medical opinion and refuse referral and treatment takes
courage, even arrogance. To act this way makes Nelson
sometimes doubt his own judgement:

◆ That decision made me feel completely responsible for my
son's illness. I was asking myself: 'What if he does have
clinical depression?' (My imagination is as lurid as the next
man's.) 'Suppose he does have anorexia and he's even more
diabolically successful at hiding it than anyone can imagine?
Perhaps he has practised and practised until he can vomit
silently?'

What finally convinced Nelson that he was right in judging
the situation for himself rather than putting his faith in
doctors was when he made a phone call to a medical colleague at work to ask for his opinion.

◆ I was utterly flabbergasted that after two minutes on the
phone he quite simply said that ME 'doesn't exist'. Our
conversation was brief. In a way it was a relief. Just as with
the psychiatrists, if he had been willing to listen to the

evidence and then delivered a considered judgement I would have been more worried. Complete prejudice, a categorical judgement delivered without hearing any of the details, at last made me realise that I was going to have to trust my own judgement because I wasn't going to get any help.

CHAPTER **11**

Alternative practitioners

We die because we are mortal, not because we are lonely
or have the wrong attitude.
DAVID SPIEGEL[1]

There is really no such thing as alternative medicine, just
medicine that works and medicine that doesn't ... There
isn't an 'alternative' physiology or anatomy or nervous
system any more than there's an alternative map of London
which lets you get to Battersea without crossing the Thames.
JOHN DIAMOND[2]

In a climate of medical incredulity and ignorance, it is not surprising that chronically ill people turn to complementary and alternative practitioners. There is a mind-blowing choice of treatments and therapies out there offering hope and salvation. In their favour, alternative therapies have emphasised the complex interplay between physical and mental well-being – a welcome antidote to the 'if-you-can't-measure-it-it-isn't-there' model of illness. This concept is now accepted to the extent that some conventionally trained doctors now offer acupuncture, homoeopathy and massage in their practices.

But have we perhaps absorbed the messages of the alternative practitioners too uncritically, and are those with ME especially vulnerable to the promises of relief or cures? With the exception of a couple of the men, everyone in my sample had made the same round of treatments, from healers to herbalists to homoeopaths, seeking validation, relief from symptoms and even a cure. The main difference between individuals was the length of their list and the limits of their belief, patience and savings.

Sifting the wheat from the chaff

In the light of the experiences reported in this book, it seems that quackery is alive and well, and it is not always easy to discriminate between this and the well-established, although not necessarily proven, ways of healing offered by trained practitioners. Peggy Munson writes of the American experience of CFIDS: 'Where medicine fails, health practitioners often make uninformed assumptions, fake knowledge, or offer pseudo-cures before admitting defeat. Contemporary society has perpetuated a tremendous number of myths about immunity, often grasping onto the persuasive language of quick-fix healing in a desperate attempt to thwart the failings of the body. Certainly true healing and quackery can happen in both allopathic and alternative medicine.'[3] Unlike conventional medicine where published clinical trials can give some guidance as to the success rate and side-effects of a particular treatment, the evaluation of alternative medicine is still in its infancy. In addition, there are those reports of an individual who claims to have been cured by a particular therapy. But one case history, one anecdote, does not count as evidence of efficacy.

How then to evaluate the myriad therapies on offer other than by the suck-it-and-see method? Reviewing the effectiveness of complementary approaches, Shepherd concludes that we should wait until alternative therapies are subjected to 'properly controlled trials' before judging whether or not they are of value.[4] His own view is that currently a few therapies may be of help, many are nonsense and a complete waste of money, and some are actually harmful, especially when a disease other than ME is missed and misdiagnosed. Stoler, reviewing a number of recent studies which supposedly proved the efficacy of alternative therapies, concluded that every single one 'either had a design flaw or showed that alternative practices had an effect that was at or below the level of placebo.'[5] Not that the placebo effect should be dismissed lightly. If body chemistry can be changed by imagining and believing that a pill, a potion or the laying on of hands works, then the placebo effect (in the sense of the power of the mind) might be a very useful tool indeed – and without the side-effects of many conventional medicines. The concept of an energy, whether from the mind or elsewhere, which can be harnessed but not measured is echoed by some of the people in this study like Janet:

◆ I thumbed my nose to all orthodox methods. It's about getting in touch with something outside of oneself, not particularly to do with any religion, but just a connection to … a tapping into a universal energy. You can get a great deal of support from that.

The conceptual straitjacket

One of the most worrying aspects of complementary therapies is that some come with conceptual straitjackets where illness may be perceived as our own fault, as a punishment, as something we do to ourselves. Such attitudes suggest that we need to be ill, that we have become ill because of our past or our personalities, or because of our way of living. The implication is that if people work on themselves, they can be cured. And if a cure remains elusive, then once again it is the fault of the individual not the therapist or the therapy.

Alison tried acupuncture for the chronic migraines which came with ME:

◆ The first thing the guy said to me, though he wrapped it up, was: 'Yes, I can give you this treatment but if it doesn't work it's not my fault, it's your fault.' Because of the way he wrapped it up, I kind of took it at first, but going away and thinking about it I thought: 'This is completely outrageous. How dare he say this.' I just stopped, I didn't go back.

Wells, writing about MS, says the same thing: 'One therapist asked me about "secondary gains", in other words what purpose illness served in my life. I searched my soul to no avail for ways in which I was using chronic illness to escape life's responsibilities or gain sympathy. I rarely seek any special dispensation for being ill; more often than not I overextend myself for fear of being considered weak or incompetent.'[6] The idea that we need to be ill is insulting and demoralising. What possible gains do people get from having ME? But this is the message which some people in the study picked up from their therapists, like Lizzie:

◆ They go, 'Well, if you do this, this and this, you'll get well.' They suggest that there is always a reason why we are ill – or that we are ill because we need to be ill.

According to this kind of philosophy, ill health arrives for a purpose and to answer some spiritual need. So, continued ill health proves only that those needs have not yet been addressed. When I was terribly ill following my relapse, one therapist told me that I 'needed' to be ill, while another said that ME was the result of an unsatisfactory relationship with my mother. I did not know what to do with these ideas.

Positive dialogues and outcomes

So far this has been a fairly negative overview of the contribution of alternative therapies but it reflects what people have said. However, negative dialogues with therapists do not form the complete picture. Three women in the sample were so drawn to a particular therapy that they started studying with a view to training themselves. None of them was 'cured' of ME, but they were helped significantly by being offered a different way of looking at the world and a different way of living. Janet now practises dowsing; May is studying alternative religions; Lizzie works as a therapist herself.

The final words in this chapter should be Lizzie's because she has wise things to say about what to take and what to leave behind. She learnt to be selective about who she consulted, learnt to take what was of value to her, and by finding the right therapist and the right therapies created a more balanced approach to her life. For her this meant tuning in not just to her fine intellect and busy mind, but also to the needs of her body by putting into practice concepts such as trying to stay grounded, judging and responding to her energy levels, and not forcing things. Through transcendental meditation and bodywork she learned:

◆ To trust something that wasn't intellectual. That bowled me over because everything had been in my mind. Something was working that was not in the mind but about energy. It was great because it threw my whole concept of what illness was about. That was good for me.

Then came a series of positive shifts from ceasing to search for a label and a cure for ME, to taking responsibility for her own health, to living with and managing her fluctuating energy levels:

◆ It feels like I'm constantly understanding more and more about what I went through and what I continue to go through during my life so I don't feel stuck on labels. The thing is I went through a lot of hard work to understand things about myself which has changed and altered my energy levels. It doesn't matter if my illness is organic or not. I've shifted things in me. I've shifted my energy levels.

So, what conclusions can we make here? Do we put faith in alternative therapies or not? The facts from this project are these: no one was cured – properly restored to full health – by any alternative therapy or complementary practitioner. Most conclude that the best they can hope for is support, help in staying on an even keel, and perhaps some relief from some symptoms. The most frequent outcome is an opportunity to develop a relationship with a wise, caring, supportive therapist who will walk with them through the ME wilderness. And for some, windows open on to a new way of dealing with health and illness, and on to different ways of living.

CHAPTER 12

Social workers and health practitioners

> I need someone who will take me in the car, who will say,
> 'Don't worry about that', who will take that stress level
> away. How am I going to get to anything if I'm not well
> enough? I need someone with me. I panic. I think: 'How
> am I going to do this?'
> DENISE

There is not a lot to say about the attitudes of social workers
and other health professionals since the majority of the
people interviewed were deemed ineligible for social work
involvement and were turned down for just about everything they applied for, including accommodation suitable
for their disabilities, home help and even visits from the
domiciliary library service. The process from start to finish
is a time-consuming and energy-wasting nightmare, as
Alison describes:

◆ The DLA [Disability Living Allowance] is a big problem
because they always assume you are lying. They say, 'We
disagree that you can't cook a main meal' and if you say you
can't, they say, 'Yes you can.' I've been cut off and gone to
tribunal. In fact, I didn't get DLA at all until I went to
tribunal. I couldn't have persevered if I hadn't had help from
an advice worker at the university. I got mobility allowance
once, and then they cut it off, and I just couldn't face
fighting for that. I feel I've had to know all about it and jump

through all the right hoops. I wouldn't have been able to
do it if I hadn't been an articulate, confident, middle-class
person with the help of this advice worker. I've had to keep
charts which are a graphic representation of how I am,
which convinced the tribunal and even the DLA finally.

Others did not want to get tangled in the maze of bureau-
cracy which would have involved energy-draining phone
calls, form filling, interviews and appeals.

The few people who did manage to work their way into
the system report very different experiences and they have
mixed views about the social workers and other support
providers who came into their lives. Phil is very positive
about the social worker to whom he turned after three years
of being cared for by his parents. When he was just well
enough to contemplate independence and knew that peace
and solitude were an absolute priority, even if it meant living
on his own for the first time in his life, he contacted a senior
social worker:

◆ Within a few weeks she'd found me this place, just like that,
through a housing association – a ground-floor flat! A home
help became part of the equation and things tied in nicely.
She was very very supportive and very helpful. I've been
here for the last six years.

The home help was a mixed blessing, proving more of a
strain than a dirty flat.

It was traumatic having a home help running about, perched
on ladders, me thinking: 'She's going to fall.' There was one
got stuck in the little shower-room, sobbing and crying to
come out. I was finding the stress of someone being here
for an hour and getting all the wrong messages more bother
than it was worth. They said they would come at 10am and
arrive at 2pm and you're lying there thinking: 'Hurry up and
get here, I need to rest.' They were well meaning, but the
home help department's knowledge of ME was less than the
GP's. I decided to do my own housework and stuff.

As his health improved, Phil took on the role of talking to
health professionals to try to educate them about ME. His
views are again very positive.

Occupational therapists, physiotherapists, nurses have been
terrific. By and large, they've wanted to learn more. It's
when I get a bit further up the tree to GPs and consultants
that I feel the doors closing.

After speaking to senior psychiatrists at the Royal Edinburgh Hospital, he asked one of the students for feedback.
'Did the psychiatrists believe him?' he asked. 'No, not one,'
was the reply.

Phil is the only person who succeeded in getting the help
he wanted. The others report negative experiences, especially
with nurses, psychiatric nurses and receptionists in doctors'
surgeries. Many struggle out of bed to talk to a psychiatric
nurse after the GP has passed the buck. Chris recalls the
response of just such a nurse to his description of his
exhaustion, constant sore throats and diarrhoea.

◆ **She said, 'It sounds like stress to me,' and gave me relaxation tapes.**

My single experience of talking to a psychiatric nurse was much the same. She was young, inexperienced, and knew nothing about ME. I had nine years' experience of it. There was no meeting point. At the end of the hour's session, I was sweating, dry-mouthed and dizzy. The nurse admitted she had nothing to offer.

Alison's experience of dealing with the social services is very different from Phil's, but more typical in terms of the attitudes she encountered. She was already ill with ME when she learnt that her mother was dying of cancer. She reports feelings of helplessness, powerless and guilt because her own illness prevented her from providing the care she longed to give. In the end, she somehow managed to travel down to be with her mother during the final six months of her life. These months proved the most testing of her long illness, but not because of her feelings of impending loss and self-recrimination for being too ill to offer more support. It was the additional physical and emotional drain of being someone with a 'mystery' illness, at a time of personal trauma, having to face hostile doctors, social workers and other health professionals:

◆ **The nurses and the social workers who came to the house didn't even seem to have heard of ME or if they had they thought of it as 'yuppie flu' or something. They did not understand my position at all and when they were talking to me, they treated me as if I was a silly, selfish, self-indulgent,**

145

irresponsible person who wasn't and couldn't be bothered to make her mother's bed. And so we got no help. Oh Jesus, it was ghastly because my mum needed me. They wouldn't listen.

Alison became embroiled for a second time with social workers out of desperation when she tried to obtain practical help and support for herself and her partner Peter – both now severely ill with ME and stranded in their fifth-floor tenement flat. This time she found herself up against another kind of block which she had not anticipated. As well as the usual negative assumptions about ME, there were also attitudes which she interpreted as class prejudice. The barriers to obtaining support and practical help proved insurmountable because the implicit assumption was that middle-class people did not turn to social services for help. The chance of a meaningful dialogue was doomed before it began.

I rang up the social work department and I sort of staggered to the door to let her in and brought her into the kitchen. It was like people in our class aren't expected to ask for home help. She sort of said that more or less, 'We don't usually give home helps to people in your situation.' I said, 'But we can't look after ourselves.'

After the interview, nothing more was heard, and Alison could not face the battle of following it up.

◆ The whole interview was so unpleasant. It was like we were
   sort of sociological specimens or just specimens that they
   were looking at. 'What are you asking for help for? You're
   not one of the class that gets helped.' I thought there was
   absolutely no point in pursuing it.

Alison also raises the controversial issue of nationality and
nationalism when she laughingly describes herself as an
obviously well-educated English woman of professional
background, a classical musician, with a maligned and misunderstood illness, asking for help with housework. She
describes the frosty and cynical reception she received.
Although she cannot prove it, she wonders if her English
accent set up yet more antagonism from the social work
department.

  While Phil dismissed his home helps because he did not
need the tension and stress which came with them, Alison
decided to pay privately for the basic help with housework
which she and her partner needed. By this time, neither was
able to work; to pay for help ate into their very limited financial resources. Despite this, Alison expresses relief at the busi-
nesslike arrangement of paying for help as opposed to
begging for it from the Department of Social Security. Paid
help brings with it no emotional baggage, no confrontations
and no hostility about ME.

◆ I discovered that you can actually pay people to help you.
   That was a tremendous boon. I started putting up notices in
   the Post Office. We've had a succession of girls – students
   – who have come up for two or three hours a week and

have done washing up and cleaning and food preparation which in a way is actually much easier to deal with, even than with very kind people helping, because it's a reciprocal thing, and so I don't have to feel so frightfully grateful to them all the time.

Throughout her interview, Denise cries out for help and support, yet after her dealings with doctors, she, and many others, cannot face any more. She carries on without support. So do the young adults – and older adults – who are cared for by their parents because they fall through the net of conditions which would have made them eligible for housing, care and mobility benefits. There is a long way to go before state-provided support, appropriate to the needs of people with ME, can be asked for without dread. Tragically, the most sick are the most defeated by the process of trying to obtain benefits and help, and so carry on without.

CHAPTER 13

Teachers

It's being shut in a room for up to two hours where the
temperature may be boiling hot in summer, or freezing cold
in winter, where the lights are flickering, and where the
ginger-headed kid at the back is spitting bits of paper
round the classroom and howling like a monkey at every
opportunity while the teacher yells at you for missing her
last lesson and not completing your homework.
JOSH

A lack of a diagnosis combined with a lingering belief
among the medical profession that children do not get ME
means that they struggle on through school long after they
should have stopped. To varying degrees, all the young
people felt pressured, hassled, threatened and bullied.
Others, keen not to be left behind, collaborated more will-
ingly in the decision to continue their education. It is testimony to the relentless pressure to keep going from doctors
and teachers that *all* the young people struggled on through
school or college long after they became ill. Six out of seven
kept going for years. All have horror stories to tell. And when
they 'failed' at school, they were at risk of being placed in
institutions such as special schools or psychiatric wards.
These are the young people's histories.

Josh attended school half-time or less, with two complete
years off, before he collapsed during Standard Grade exams.
By this time he could hardly get out of bed in the morning,

let alone move from classroom to classroom, concentrate on eight different subjects, or cope with the bedlam of the breaks and lunchtimes. He describes life at the local comprehensive as 'absolute hell', an ordeal he has paid for ever since. Since the age of 15, he has been housebound and profoundly ill.

Rachel was forced through school after she became ill at the age of 11. She was then placed in a series of totally inappropriate institutions, including a treatment centre for emotionally disturbed children, a special residential school, an infectious diseases ward, and an adult HIV and drug rehab ward.

By the time she was 10, Ruby was too ill to attend school but she and her mother were 'constantly harassed' about her falling attendance so, for six months more, she struggled on while vomiting blood and fainting in and outside the classroom. Her mother tried and failed to negotiate with the school. She was eventually accused of Munchhausen's syndrome by proxy.

Kirsty attended school for two years after she became ill, always feeling unwell, but somehow got through her Standard Grade exams. Then, despite deteriorating health, she continued with her Highers. Then it was 'down, and further down.' In the end, Kirsty was bedbound for two years.

David struggled through school from the age of 7, attending part-time, until a major relapse brought him to a halt at the age of 14. He was bedbound for four years. Now 22, he has never resumed his education, nor can he work.

Jessie struggled through secondary school for two years after becoming ill aged 12. Then, as her health deteriorated, she collected work and did it at home. She sat Standard Grade and Higher examinations at home, and managed a year at Heriot-Watt University. A year into her degree course, she became too ill to continue her studies. She is now back home.

Chris, like Jessie, somehow managed to keep going – two years at college to get his HND followed by a three-year degree course at Edinburgh University – but the price now is chronic ill health. Chris has been housebound for two years.

Here is evidence of young people paying the price of putting education before their health. Teachers and doctors need to be educated about ME so that they understand that when a young person is pushed beyond their energy limits, the consequences can be catastrophic.

The school environment can be harsh and brutal for someone who is feeling ill. The physical demands of climbing up flights of stairs, traipsing the crowded corridors, hanging around the playground in the cold, walking from building to building can exhaust even fit young people. But for children with ME school is a nightmare of physical, mental and sensory overload. Kirsty describes it as:

◆ Exceptionally difficult. Even carrying a bag. I mean we used to have to bring our whole books in for the day and carry them about with us all day. Even that, little things like that, were really a struggle.

At lunchtime, when energy levels hit rock bottom, what do these sick children do? At Josh's 1000-place comprehensive school, the canteen could only accommodate a hundred pupils at a time, so:

◆ The only option was to take to the streets in search of a
chippy where you had to stand for half an hour in a queue
before running back to school in order not to miss the bell
and be put on detention.

Several of the young people I interviewed were so physically
and emotionally stressed by the school environment, that it
literally made them vomit. Ruby threw up regularly. Josh
frequently developed a migraine, and on one occasion threw
up all over his friend when the teacher refused to let him out
of the room to get a drink of water.

If the physical environment is hard, the intellectual
demands are often impossible with the 'brain-fog' aspect of
ME going unrecognised and unacknowledged. Young people
with ME are expected to jump through the same hoops as
the other pupils, produce work on time and concentrate in
lessons, even though their brains are screaming for release. It
is difficult to adequately describe the agony they must go
through as they try to learn in such uncompromising conditions. No one would demand the same of a child with any
other serious health problem. Jessie, highly motivated,
describes how difficult it was to keep going:

◆ My memory and concentration got worse and worse. It got
to the point where I remember sitting reading my chemistry
books and I was reading the same passage again and again
and it wasn't going in. And at that point I was ready to
crack. The fact that I couldn't work really upset me.

Every aspect of the school environment is difficult for a young person with ME but the worst, as Josh describes, is the total lack of control:

◆ You are herded like cattle. You may need to lie down, need to go to the toilet, need something to eat because your blood sugar is low, need the glaring fluorescent light turned off, but instead the physics teacher is shouting at you, 'Why don't you understand this? It's so simple? Why have you not done your homework? Everybody else has.'

Should these ill young people be in a classroom at all?

Not being believed

For all the young people, the most painful part of coping with ME in school was not being believed (*see also* pages 120–34). Still naïve enough to believe in a just and fair world – at least at the start of their illnesses – these young people were aghast that adults refused to accept their accounts of how they felt. It was a shock to find out that when faced with a tearful and distressed child, grown-ups were rude, ignorant and dismissive. As time went on, the young people grew wise and cynical and their expectations of adults plummeted. Even Kirsty, a gentle young woman, concludes of her teachers, 'They were ignorant.'

All the young people who took part in this project spontaneously said that they had been accused of 'skiving'. All documented confrontations with teachers in which they felt that their illness was thrown back in their faces as trivial, imagined or an excuse for not working. Before ME, Kirsty threw herself into life inside and out of the classroom. She was no slouch:

◆ Every night of the week was busy. I played hockey, played badminton once a week, went to an aerobics class once a week, helped out with Brownies once a week and the Anchor Boys once a week. Then I helped my elderly aunt with MS and also a part-time job at a newsagents.

So why should this girl suddenly become a 'skiver' as her teachers suggested? When she was away for almost a year, both teachers and pupils assumed she was pregnant and had taken time off to have a baby, something she relates with grim humour:

◆ And I thought: 'Some chance.' I had no social life, you know. I thought it would be easier to have a baby and, you know, you'd have a product after being ill say for maybe nine months. You had a product at the end of the day.

Angry words, angry behaviour

Instead of sympathy, young people find themselves on the receiving end of anger and aggression from teachers who dislike their classroom routines and timetables disrupted by illness. Pupils who failed to achieve decent grades through absence and illness were made to feel guilty and worthless. They were told they were failing their teachers and letting down their school. The anger expressed by teachers is a reflection of a mind-set that education only happens between the ages of 5 and 18, inside the four walls of the classroom, and that every day of the timetable missed is a minor catastrophe. The assumption is that school is the most important event in any young person's life. Josh describes a 'full-blown military enforcement' of the curriculum and an intolerable build-up of pressure during the exam years, with comments like:

- 'This is the most important day of your life.'
- 'You have to come to school more often or there will be repercussions.'
- 'You'll be a binman if you fail these exams.'
- 'If you could be bothered to come to school more often you wouldn't be so far behind with your work.'

As Josh got more and more behind with his exam work, his teachers took his absence as a personal affront:

- It was seen as an insult to their authority. You could see their rage and anger.

Kirsty too was constantly told off by teachers who regarded her absence as a dereliction of duty:

- I will make an appointment and you will come and see me and you will do this and you will do that.

It is revealing that Jessie, the only young person who managed to keep up with her exam subjects by going into school for a few hours a week to collect and give back her work, received the least hassle from her teachers. She describes their attitude to her unusual regime as 'accepting' rather than intolerant because she delivered. She was able to fulfil the role they expected of her and so they left her alone. She even got some help from one or two individuals.

> I didn't get the most positive reaction from teachers. No. The school weren't falling over themselves to help me. But there again, I put in the effort and they were quite obliging. My guidance teacher set up a system so I could sign in and out even though I was too young to do that, so he helped me a lot.

Jessie was fortunate in having a few teachers who already knew people with ME. This seems to be crucial. For children and adults alike, personal experience of ME is a key which opens doors of support and understanding. Jessie was just well enough to satisfy the school and maintain her own high standards of academic work. Others were too ill to keep going. Unlike Jessie, they were neither accepted nor tolerated.

A culture of blame

The culture of blaming the ill for their own misfortune spills over into the school environment. Teachers blame children and young people with ME, making them feel guilty in ways which would be unthinkable with other recognised illnesses. It is always the child's fault that they are ill, and illness is reinvented as optional behaviour. The most commonly reported remark from teachers in the transcripts is, 'This is unacceptable behaviour.' Josh's guidance teacher would regularly call him to her room and say:

◆ Well, what does your doctor say? I want a letter from your doctor. I want a letter saying you can't do your homework.

But since the doctor did not believe him either, no letter was forthcoming and the exhausting game played on.

Like the teachers, healthy children do not understand ME, and they have other agendas. Why should they? Children can be cruel – it is a fact of life that they pick on the weakest, the fattest, the thinnest, the one with glasses. Young people who attend school part-time, who turn up for an hour or two then go home or who spend time in the sick room, are simply weird. They are wimps. All the young people in this study suffered from the bullying and taunting of their peers. What is astounding is that the teachers sided with the bullies, blaming the sick kids for upsetting and disrupting peer relationships. Josh recalls a teacher telling him:

◆ You're upsetting the other pupils by not coming to school. No wonder they pick on you. If you could be bothered coming to school more often, you wouldn't be hassled by the other kids.

When teachers are bullies

Each young person I interviewed had at least one horror story to relate. Whether coincidentally or not, each one involved either a Guidance, Learning Support or PE teacher. One can only speculate why these particular members of staff were cruel and incredulous and came up with wildly inappropriate and counterproductive behaviours in response to a child telling them they were too ill to work or do sport.

In one of the transcripts there is a classic metaphor of the sick person shut away out of sight where she cannot offend or upset others. Here is the mad, bad young woman removed from mainstream society and shut away. Kirsty gives us this image when she describes her Learning Support teacher's response to a request for help. When she could no longer cope with a full school day, she was offered a dark cupboard as a sick room. What upset her was not so much the claustrophobic cupboard as the way she was made to feel about using it:

◆ She was Head of Learning Support. I went down to see her, you know, to try and find something I could maybe do and adjust my timetable and she said, 'Well, you could just come and do some work with me and then if you felt tired you could just sit in this wee cupboard here and bring a teabag in your pocket and sit there.' It was a tiny wee cupboard. You know, it was like I was just a bit tired and there was nothing physically wrong with me that I should be put in this wee cupboard. I felt like a naughty schoolgirl.

When my eldest son was ill with ME, he told me an apocryphal (but not unusual) tale about his mate who also had ME. The two of them were attending school part-time, had taxis to ferry them there and back, and collapsed on their beds when they arrived home. Every week the PE teacher would ask for a note to excuse them from PE, never believing that the boys were seriously ill. In his eyes, they were a pair of feeble skivers. Andrew forgot his note one week, and being a gentle soul – as well as a very ill one – did not put up a fight. The PE teacher found a pair of outsize shorts and made him run twice around the perimeter of the playing fields. The consequences for Andrew were an extreme exacerbation of symptoms and several months in bed.

An unequal dialogue

Children and young people usually know a lot more about ME than their teachers but are unable to talk to them about their illness when their status in school vetoes any kind of meaningful dialogue. It may be that the school environment militates against teachers acknowledging ignorance or permitting themselves to be in the position of learners – less knowledgeable and less experienced than the children they teach. The explicit and implicit rule of the classroom is that teachers know more than their pupils. Many teachers, influenced by the negative attitudes of the medical profession and the media, may already 'know' all about ME. They know that it is an excuse for idleness and something which is 'all in the mind'. How do children talk to teachers who are not predisposed to listen and not inclined to believe?

Some young people want to remain at school because they are happy there, but if they do decide to carry on, it must be on their own terms, and with the support, tolerance and understanding of the staff. And any such arrangement must be regarded as an achievement not a failure. They need kind words – and somewhere quiet to go when they are done in.

Each and every one of the young people who struggle on through school with ME deserves a medal. They deserve awards for courage and bravery for just being there at all.

CHAPTER 14

Family and friends

*If only you would embrace Jesus and let him into your
heart, you would get better.*
JOSH'S GRANDMOTHER

ME is a lonely illness. Some people are so ill that they exist
for years cut off from the outside world, too ill to communicate with friends and family, even by telephone. Others, not
quite poleaxed, surface occasionally as if from underground
to glimpse the light of day before being buried in illness
once again. Most of the moderately ill try to pass for normal
some of the time, keeping the true extent of their suffering
to themselves.

Alison and Peter, a couple with ME, were isolated 84 steps
up in the top flat of a Victorian tenement. They describe
their way of life in a way which is almost funny – almost:

◈ **There wasn't really anyone to tell. We kind of survived on
carry-outs from the Chinese takeaway, and Indian deliveries.**

Keeping the larder minimally stocked involved lowering a
basket on the end of a long rope which the local grocer would
fill, then hoisting the load back up the stairwell. They did not
seek help from other people on the communal stair because
they were too ill to cope with the necessary introductions and
explanations.

ME changes friends into people with peculiar behaviour patterns. Janet says that during the years of her illness, the most she could cope with was limited one-to-one interaction. Even now she finds a lot of talking exhausting and has to tailor her social activities to her limited energy levels. And this after seventeen years.

> I still like having family parties. I like having people in for meals but I have to make it lunch now because I'm whacked by 7.30pm.

Chloe weeps in her interview when she describes her isolation. For her, and for Denise and Mike, the prospect of identical days of solitude, stretching as far as the eye can see, housebound in a small flat, is intolerable. Loneliness also comes from attempts to protect others from the reality of ME by trying to pass now and again for normal. Friends see the short burst of normal activity, but they do not see the collapse afterwards. As a friend wrote after just such as effort, 'I am in penalty time now.' Chloe chides herself for putting on an act for others, but sees no alternative if she wants company:

> They don't really see you at your worst because when they see you, you've made an effort and you've put on your make-up, you've done your hair, you've changed your clothes, and you've done nothing all day to get the wee bit of energy to go to a friend's house. They say, 'You look great. You're sounding great.' They don't realise that if I have a late night, say I'm at friends, I'll come back, I'm ill the

next good few days. You can be ill for the week. They don't see that. That's the difficulty. I try to explain to them and they try to take it on board but they don't understand.

Lizzie, although not so ill, reports the same dilemma:

◆ I had friends who maybe pulled away and got confused because I'd be fine when I was with them, I'd have lots of energy, and then I'd go home and I'd be … phew!

The loss of a social structure is a big part of the erosion of the quality of life. Everyone talked about isolation – one called it 'a life sentence' – an isolation born again and again out of others' misperceptions and misunderstanding, an interminable, soul-destroying isolation.

So what are the attitudes of those closest to people with ME? Family and friends observe for themselves the struggles and the pain, yet according to the stories told here, while some are accepting and believing, many more are not.

While individual accounts differ, in the common pool of experience there are several dominant themes. Gender differences are marked. Most (but not all) men get less flack than women and children, and are more likely to be believed. Men are brave, women are feeble, children are skivers. Relatives and friends cope better with those who are brave, stoic and silent. They are less supportive towards those who are emotionally needy, who seek sympathy and talk a lot about their illness. Friends and colleagues of long standing are more supportive than recent acquaintances. As a result, people with ME need to monitor the attitudes of those close to them, picking up the good vibes and the bad, because they do not have the energy to deal with a difficult father, sister-in-law or friend who has the power to demean them.

The men who are not floored by ME

Six out of the seven men are fairly positive about relatives and friends. However, they are also fairly reticent and do not warm to the subject as do the women. While they talk at length and with emotion about the impact of ME on their wives, partners and children, they barely mention other family members. Other topics engage them – such as the struggle to keep working and the attitudes of the medical world. What they do say, however, is significant: they choose not to talk about their illness, preferring to keep it to themselves, and so do not offer any hostages to fortune. By not seeking sympathy, they do not risk rejection. By underplaying the impact of their illness on the quality of their life, they do not invite crass comments. This behaviour says as much about families as about the men who are ill since it seems that those who are near and dear cannot necessarily be trusted to cope with the reality of the illness.

With the exception of their wives, Liam and Alistair say almost nothing about those close to them. Liam is more preoccupied with maintaining 'a healthy department' than worrying about individual responses to ME, and he copes with his illness by retreating into solitude. Alistair laughs off the dismissive attitudes of his colleagues in the surgery, putting their lack of sympathy down to their own stress levels. Fraser, Ray and Mike talk almost as one; they avoid the subject of their illness whenever possible and so do not invite any kind of response. Mike says:

◆ I don't discuss it a lot. I just say, 'Oh I'm all right. I'm fine.' I just sort of sweep it under the carpet. I don't think they'd be too interested if I started going on and on, 'Oh, I don't feel well.' No, I tend to deal with it myself.

Even when visiting his sister, he refuses to let his illness intrude. While she is aware that he is not well, it is not something they discuss. Mike seems content with this strategy saying:

◆ There have been no problems at all.

The men are in general tolerant of those who fail to appreciate the extent of their disabilities and seem to cope well, even with teasing and indifference which would possibly reduce many women to tears. Fraser describes the 'usual banter' down at the rugby club:

◆ You know the sort of humour you get in a rugby club. Because I didn't have a black eye or was in plaster or stitches, nobody could really work out why I wasn't playing and training. I was trying to tell them how I was feeling and they would just get giggly, you know. But they weren't being nasty about it. They didn't know … they didn't appreciate what was going on … Oh, I didn't get upset about it because I knew the guys before this came along … it was just, you know, a few beers and a bit of a laugh. If anybody was unsympathetic, it was only because they hadn't heard of it, or they couldn't understand why I wasn't feeling well because I looked OK.

At the fire station, the tone was much the same:

◆ I can't remember any hostility to be quite honest with you. Apart from the general banter and a bit of carry-on. After a while I told them what the score was and of course it was met with a load of hilarity. That's the sort of black humour you get at the fire service because it has to be that way.

Fraser is content to leave it there. He chooses, like the others, not to waste energy trying to explain. Maybe Fraser accepts this lack of interest and empathy because he is never terribly ill. Maybe he is a macho bloke who expects nothing more. Or maybe he knows that to pursue explanations of his illness would be completely pointless:

◆ Well, I knew that as soon as I tried to put my cards on the table and tried to be serious with them, I knew what the reaction would be. I knew it would be a load of stick. I was expecting that anyway. But eventually the jokes subsided.

This suited Fraser. It was part of his survival strategy.

◆ I didn't look for anyone to lean on. I still wanted to be treated the same.

The men attribute the lack of real nastiness to the fact that prior to becoming ill they were known and respected as active, healthy people, doing jobs and playing sport and engaging in community activities. The change was therefore obvious and there was a baseline for comparison. But, as Ray says, new acquaintances are a different matter:

People who've known me a long time, they know how I do things. If I'm complaining of something all the time then they know there's something amiss here. The problems are with people who haven't known me for very long.

And although Fraser is teased at the rugby club – and takes it in good spirit – he knows that he *would* be believed if anyone felt like challenging him:

Because I was playing rugby and I was a fireman and had a macho kind of background, people thought: 'Well, there must be something wrong with him if it's going on as long as this.' … of course, my close circle of friends knew that it wasn't me, you know, they knew that something was wrong and were quite supportive from the start.

Yet ME is not acknowledged as a serious, disabling illness for the men – although at first glance this may seem to be the case. While avoiding discussing ME and tending to make light of their disabilities may be the best strategy for them, their reticence does others no favours. By remaining quiet, these stoic men maintain the taboo and push the illness, and those who suffer from it, further underground, reinforcing the attitudes of the medical profession that anyone who complains is a whinger. Perhaps doctors and teachers would take ME seriously if men like Fraser and Liam and Mike and Alistair made more of a noise about it. But the pressure on men to be stoic in the face of adversity is strong in our society. It is not their fault that they choose to keep their suffering to themselves. And as everyone – women and young people included – said in their interviews, there comes a point in this long illness when you tire of explaining the unexplainable, as Fraser says:

◆ You can only repeat something so much. I mean, 'How are you feeling this morning?' and it's the same story as a week ago, yesterday, a fortnight ago, a month ago, you know. Nothing changes. I was fed up with telling everyone the story of what I might possibly have. I had to go into this whole, 'ME? What's that?' and you had to go into this whole sort of spiel about what you thought was wrong. It got wearing after a while. Oh aye, it would have been easier wearing a badge.

Seriously ill men

The option of passing for healthy – or at least not revealing the full extent of the suffering imposed by ME – is not possible for two of the men. They are too beaten by ME to collude in any pretence about its severity, or put on a brave smile in order to make life easier for those close to them. Their illness is blatantly obvious, yet despite having a similar level of disability, the stories they tell about those close to them could not be more different.

Phil, who rated himself 90 per cent disabled at his worst, was so ill that in his late twenties he had to return home to be cared for by his parents. In a claustrophobic atmosphere, among boisterous younger siblings, there was no hiding his suffering, but although it was not an easy option – and tensions often ran high – they pulled through:

◆ They took me back with open arms. Out of concern.

Phil's friends also stuck by him, and for the same reason the other men cite:

◆ I mean, I'm talking about my mates that I've known since childhood who could see such a radical transformation. They could see more than the doctors because they were seeing me on a day-to-day basis. They knew I was the one who didn't want to leave the disco until four in the morning and would be out running at eight. They saw me going from that to a timid wreck, barely able to drink. They could see that and they knew that something was badly wrong – when the doctors were talking about withdrawal from the world, depression and the psychology of illness. I knew who to put my trust in. I knew who was really listening, who could really see what was going on.

Jamie, on the other hand, has a tough time of it. Neither one of the walking wounded, just well enough to pass for normal some of the time, nor so catastrophically ill that he is unable to care for himself, he seems to be in the worst possible situation. Of his family, he says:

They were the worst. My mother went into a real panic and was unpleasant about it. She said quite clearly she wouldn't let my illness hold her back ... I have a sister and she was just bloody hopeless.

Jamie was stuck with two choices. Either he cut himself off from close relatives who had forced him into a defensive position by questioning the validity of his illness, or he embarked on a long battle to convince them and win them round. He chose the latter course with his mother, navigating through difficult and fundamental changes in his relationship with her:

I just had to be clear, which was something I had never done to her before. I said, 'Look, if you act like this, I won't ever plan to come so you won't see me at all. You've got to accept this is how I am, and I'll come and see you only when I can.'

Things worked out – but only over a very long period, and with a lot of work on Jamie's part in psychotherapy sessions.

Friends were no better. They failed to grasp how terribly ill Jamie was, preferring to brush the whole thing off. He relates the following encounter in which a close friend tells him how he feels and how he should deal with his illness:

He thought it best to help me deny it, so I had to become more assertive. The crunch came when he tried to jolly me along. I told him to leave. He didn't believe me so I told him to fuck off. That was a strong thing to do but it helped me then.

This need to monitor the reactions of others is expressed by many of the interviewees. Like others, Jamie talks of the need to protect himself by not getting embroiled in painful arguments and explanations with people who try to jolly him along and who trivialise his suffering:

◆ I am overly noticing of people who don't ask, or ask in a way that's not going to give them any trouble – you know, having to do anything or having to feel sorry for me. I don't want that.

As with others, he finds sympathy and understanding from people who knew him in a professional capacity and in a context where his reputation and his contribution to society were known and acknowledged prior to illness:

◆ I get a lot of personal support from the local history society. I invested a lot of my time there. People stop me in the street and say very kindly, 'We really miss you,' and, 'Things are not the same without you.'

In this, Jamie is like the other men who were able to carry on working. In contexts in which people with ME previously had strong identities, and where they were known and respected, the healthy do not try to play the amateur psychologist. The evidence is that people with ME can be themselves – their ill selves – most comfortably among those with whom they have already worked or played.

Women's friends and families

Unlike the men, the women became deeply engrossed in this subject. They were discursive, eloquent, analytic, thankful, puzzled, tearful and angry about the attitudes and behaviour of relatives and friends who responded unpredictably to their illness. They reported a much wider range of experiences than the men, from loving support to painful silence to complete disregard for their suffering. While Alison, Chloe and Lizzie talked with gratitude about the kindness and support which came from their immediate families, Denise and Janet, both severely affected, reported belittling and hostile attitudes. Fiona said that there were splits within her family: while her parents were 'very good and very understanding', extended family members thought her illness was psychological. May, like most of the men, chose not to lean on her family, preferring to deal with her illness herself.

Compared with the men, the women had higher expectations of their friends and relatives, hoping, especially in the early stages of their illness, for compassion, concern and help. They expected parents, siblings, in-laws and close friends to observe the changes imposed by ME and to attribute those changes to the ravages of a serious, physical illness. They looked for practical help and emotional support but, like Janet, they have had to come to terms with a very different reality:

◆ There was a sort of blank wall from all of them. I think they probably thought it was a neurotic reaction.

In the past, these women often played a caring role, whether as a mother, a daughter or a friend, and so when support falls away, as it did for Chloe and Denise, they feel terribly let down:

◆ I've been a true friend. I'm usually there for my friends but sometimes I wonder just how much they care about me.

Denise is equally hurt and baffled by the reaction of her friends:

◆ I'm one of those people that everyone comes to – you know everybody comes to me with their problems. It's hard when I can't get help with my problems and with this illness. Hardly anyone phones. I had a girlfriend – this is very sad – she used to get angry with me, 'Come on, we'll go to the shops.' We'll do this and that. And I would say, 'I can't, I can't walk, I'm really not feeling well.' See – they saw me as they always do. She said, 'You must try.' But I couldn't.

While some receive support from a few close contacts, others are shocked that even a sister or a flatmate shows not the slightest sympathy or understanding. Denise is hurt and baffled by her family's pretence that she is not really ill. Over and over again she says what a world of difference some practical help and understanding would have made to the quality of her life. But her family entered into a conspiracy of rejection, refusing to help and treating her as if she were still well, or at least only trivially ill:

◆ I've felt very much on my own and at times I've thought I can't go on … If only my family would just say, 'Can I give you a hand?' But they don't want to know. In fact my sister said to my mum, 'I'm not going to bother phoning her because that's all we hear from her.'

While refusing sympathy, this sister continues to make demands on the obliging Denise with requests for a manicure or a massage, while her mother chides her to pull herself together.

For most of the women, friends were worse than family. Support was not there. Friends did not try to understand the life changes imposed by ME and tended to dismiss the illness as trivial, psychological and boring. Even minimum contact – a phone call or brief visits – ceased as friends remained oblivious to the difference which a small gesture of support would have made. Chloe weeps when she says of her friends:

◆ They have not been there for me.

Denise, Janet and Alison coped with years of solitude. Janet says her friends 'switched off'. Fiona says:

◆ There was no contact. They just fell away.

A couple of the women behave like the men by presenting a stoic front and hiding the full extent of their pain and disability. They do not seek support nor try to change attitudes. They do not tell it how it is. This is one way of deflecting disappointment and dealing with a very difficult illness. Like most of the men, Janet expected little and received little:

◆ Nothing was known about it. I'm not the sort of person who likes to talk about how I feel anyway, so I usually say, 'I'm fine,' and leave it at that.

May also avoided people:

◆ I found I could not talk to anyone really close, my mother, my in-laws ... I needed to talk to someone who was sort of a friend but not too close a friend. I couldn't speak to anyone I was closely involved with without bursting into tears. And I couldn't explain. I longed to curl up in a little corner and have nothing to do with anyone.

This is the response of an ill woman who recognises that she is too emotionally fragile to cope with someone opening the floodgates of her agony and despair.

All the women were judged implicitly or explicitly by some of their relatives and friends to be suffering from a psychological illness. Denise is told by her mother and sister to pull herself together. Ruth, in extreme pain for 24 hours a day, says of her entire family:

◆ They want to get at my secret psychological problem. If only I would see the right psychologist, my illness would go away.

Yet the women are surprisingly tolerant of the psychobabble offered by family and friends. The impact on Fiona was that she started to believe she had a psychological problem herself; yet still she makes allowances for them:

◆ I felt pretty bad about myself because I was doing this big guilt thing thinking it was psychological. I kept it hidden because most of us tend to put a bright face on things … It must have been incredibly difficult for them because if you see somebody with a broken leg, then you know there's a cause and there's a time limit, but with ME you don't really see anything physical apart from, you know, they're not right and they're tired. I'm sure it causes conflicting emotions if people visit and think: 'Is it all in her head?' It is very difficult to understand. It is very difficult for members of the family to understand.

Another kind of tolerance is to acknowledge, as Denise does, that other people's lives are already too crowded to make room for someone with ME. Cindy goes further, saying that all of us walk through life, with or without ME, with only a small number of people who truly care until finally we understand the positive side of solitude:

◆ There are very few people in life who will understand you anyway, whether you've got an illness or not, and I've realised that more and more. It's like: 'How many people in your lifetime really know who you are, or care, or really know what you're going through?'

When I asked her if it was a waste of time trying to make people understand, she said:

◆ It's brilliant when you really start to clock that because it's like you don't waste energy. You're left with solitude and one or two people who understand. I think that's what life is about most of the time anyway. Your solitude can be a way of having a better relationship with yourself.

Young people and their friends

The erstwhile friends of children and young people with ME are most noticeable by their absence. While a child may get a bit of sympathy and some good-natured teasing about a leg in plaster, a child with ME can expect only incomprehension – or worse. Some were taunted by their friends; others were physically and verbally abused inside and outside the classroom.

Children who are ill have the hardest time with their peers during their primary school years and in the first years of secondary school when children are intolerant of anyone who is different, weak or vulnerable. The child with ME becomes a scapegoat and an easy target for school bullies. Jessie, confident and self-possessed despite her experiences of illness, talks about the 'snide comments' she got when she was younger:

◆ I didn't really get bullied or anything, but the comments really hurt, you know. I didn't like it at all. I hated people thinking I was a skiver.

The snide comments were particularly wide of the mark in her case because she was putting so much effort into trying to keep up with her work – to the exclusion of all other activities and any social life. What hurt her was the fact that it cost her dearly in terms of increased symptoms and isolation, to achieve what her peers managed with considerably less effort:

◆ It does bother you to think people think you are having an easy time and you're not – you're really ill, you know. The hard thing was that when I was in school I'd channel all my energy for the day into those couple of lessons, so I'd seem OK, and people couldn't understand that I was ill because I looked fine. That was one of the hardest things.

It still hurts me more than I can express to hear my own son recall how every week at primary school, in the changing room before PE, he was kicked in the shins while all the kids chanted 'skiver' because he could not run or swim or take part in team games without becoming totally exhausted. And still he tried. He would kick the ball around the pitch or run about the gym, returning home ashen, in pain and beaten.

Ruby believes that her friends deserted her not because they thought she was feeble and a skiver, but because they were frightened of hurting her:

◆ I think they were a bit scared of me because they thought if they touched me I would break into a thousand pieces. They kind of thought I was too sick to do anything and to come outside. I was all fragile.

At first glance, this suggests that some children are more tolerant of illness than others, and perhaps more frightened by it. Or is it possible that Ruby's description of her friends' fear that she would break into a thousand pieces reflects how she herself felt, rather than how they felt about her. Alternatively – and this is relevant for everyone with ME – the explanation for her friends' fearful rather than hostile reaction may lie in the visibility of her symptoms which were particularly florid, with episodes of 'conking out on the floor' and 'blood pouring out of my mouth'. She reports that teachers wanted to take her to A & E. So here, instead of the invisible symptoms which most young people bring with them into the classroom and playground, was evidence of a 'real' illness which produces a different, more sympathetic and practical response from peers and teachers alike.

Older children are perhaps more tolerant – or maybe they lose interest in picking on the weakest. Instead of being bullied and tormented, the young person with ME is marginalised or ignored. In the middle years of secondary school, peer groups develop, each with its own image, attitudes and behaviours.[1,2] Boys and girls embedded in such tight-knit groups may be less aware of – or less interested in – others who do not attract or interest them. Jessie says things got easier as she moved through secondary school, and in the sixth form rules were relaxed, the timetable became more flexible, pupils were treated in a more grown-up way, and she no longer stuck out like a sore thumb. She was no longer a pariah because 'everyone wandered in and out for lessons.' Finally, she faded into the background.

The sense of loss and desolation is almost tangible as the young people talk about the way their friends gave up on them. At this critical stage of social development when the peer group makes the world go round, adolescents with ME languish at home with only their parents and their pets for friends. For some there is virtually no contact with people of their own age. This loss on their developing self-identity and confidence can only be devastating, as they watch their friends pass on through the sexually aware and wildly experimenting teenage years, then leave home – free to go to college or university. They describe a loneliness of a heart-breaking kind.

The loss of the chance to grow up

At a superficial level being ill during the teenage years is about missing out on the normal activities of adolescence such as games of football and evenings at the pub. But it is much more than that. It is about missing the chance to develop socially, to make relationships, to develop a sense of identity and to find out who you are. It is about growing up, as Jessie is well aware:

◆ I think it's a shame for any young person to be ill because you are missing out on so much stuff. I suppose when you are an adult you are still missing out on stuff, but it's not the kind of growing up bit, is it?

This is exactly it. Young people with ME are denied the opportunity to grow up. Instead, they watch their peers move on socially and academically while they remain stuck – growing older, growing wiser – but not moving on at all.

The young people understand this. They know that their losses are both superficial and very deep. Chris talks about getting through his degree courses but to the exclusion of all interaction with his peers:

◈ Basically, that was all I did. I was going to lectures and coming home again. No social life except from what was maybe in the classes. Missing out. There was all this social interaction and I was missing out on it.

Jessie says the same:

◈ All the socialising, making friends, and going out in big groups, going drinking, going clubbing and all the things which at that age I didn't do. That's the main thing I missed out on really, the social side of things. I resent the illness taking that away from me.

And Kirsty:

◈ I've missed an awful lot. Just even going out to clubs and pubs. Not that I enjoy pubs that much, but just things like that, you know, just doing normal regular things. I suppose having it [ME] younger, or if you'd had it older, say maybe in your thirties, it wouldn't have been quite so bad. But because I suppose you're still growing, developing at the age of 15 or 16, you're still trying to find yourself and find your feet in life.

The young people all talked about the paradox of feeling both older and younger than their peers, socially immature yet, like children who have endured more than their share of suffering, old beyond their years. Kirsty says:

◆ Sometimes, for a while, I thought I had matured and then suddenly I thought: 'Well, maybe I'm not matured.' Part of me has matured but another part is still young.

In their exploration of experience and feeling, they revealed insight, wisdom, compassion and humanity that was unusual for people of their age. No doubt, isolation forced them to rely heavily on their inner resources, and for some, years of being bedbound and housebound gave them more than enough time to reflect on their own and others' experiences. Jessie says:

◆ I think it makes you grow up as well, which is sad. I think I'm more self-sufficient perhaps. I think it gives you an empathy with other people going through similar things. It makes you grow up a lot when you are still young. You don't have the same opportunities to just act your age. You are weighed down by illness. It's hard. Yeah.

Put another way, what is lost is the opportunity to make choices. Maybe going to pubs and clubs, getting drunk, staying up all night and having a wild time would not have been everyone's choice of activity, but, as Josh says, he wanted the chance to choose or reject that option for himself. And all the other options which were denied him. Chris, like Josh, regards this as his greatest loss:

◆ Control. Control of my body and control over making choices. I've had the choices taken away.

No boyfriends, no girlfriends

Young people with ME are denied another very significant part of growing up – forming and experimenting with their first and early sexual relationships. From about the age of 12 or 13, the time when young people start secondary school, the fantasies and realities of non-platonic relationships dominate young people's lives. This is an exciting, difficult, demanding and heart-pounding time, but while the healthy individuals meet at night in the park and get off with one another at parties, many young people with ME grow up not knowing what it is like to have a boyfriend or girlfriend. It may be that they are so frequently absent from school, and knocked out by part-time attendance, that they have nothing left for a relationship with someone special. For others, a close relationship falls apart because they lack the physical and emotional stamina needed to sustain it. It is almost impossible, given the uniquely disabling and unpredictable nature of ME, for young people to form and sustain relationships with the opposite sex. For a long time Jessie kept her relationship with her boyfriend going by negotiating a 'long-distance' arrangement. She saw him about once a month:

◆ It was all I could deal with. That was enough. It's all I had the energy for.

But for the others there is disappointment, heartbreak or nothing. Josh struggled for a year with an intense and difficult relationship with a girl who had her own problems before he admitted that the relationship was causing his health to deteriorate further. In the end he withdrew, but he was haunted by the break-up for years afterwards. Kirsty became emotionally involved with a boy while she was still ill. The eighteen months it lasted were wonderful after the childlike existence of being confined at home. The relationship boosted her sense of self and made her feel good about herself:

◆ We just got on so well. Brilliantly as friends. And then it did progress into more than friends. It was really good.

But things went wrong. He started to 'put her down', pointing out her inadequacies as she bent over backwards to try to live up to his expectations and pass for normal. After he moved away, travelling to see him was too much for her. Despite saving up all her money to visit him, knocking herself out with each trip, spending a fortune on phone calls, in the end the relationship 'fizzled out'. The strain on both of them was too much. There were floods of tears as Kirsty talked about the loss of her boyfriend:

◆ It's like a bereavement. I thought that was a normal part – even though it was long distance – it was a normal part of life.

With the loss of her boyfriend, her self-confidence crashed. While this young man was there for her, she felt good about herself. But her self-esteem was too fragile to hold up after the break-up, so Kirsty is left once more with her illness, isolation and nothing but her memories to remind her that for a while she was a normal, attractive young woman.

For others, there is not even a taste of the roller-coaster of longing, love and rejection. Chris has recently met someone he is attracted to, but asks himself how on earth he is supposed to manage a relationship while he is so ill:

◆ Who want to impose restrictions on someone else? You know, it's like: 'Yes I could go out with you but I couldn't do this and I couldn't do that.' It's bad enough when you let yourself down without letting someone else down. I just can't imagine why anyone would hitch up with ... I've had this conversation with other people as well ... who would hitch up with some who's so disabled? Of course, people do. But I just think I couldn't.

These are the unique disabilities of ME which overwhelm and dominate each individual to the extent that no spontaneity and forward planning is possible. Under these conditions, most intimate relationships falter and fade leaving young people with their loneliness and their memories.

PART 3

Relationships

CHAPTER **15**

How couples cope

ME gets in the way of everything including relationships.
I have mixed feelings about the fact it's over. Part of me
is extremely sad. Part of me is enjoying being able to be
selfish again.

PHIL on the break-up of a five-year relationship

Two adults remained unattached throughout their illnesses.
Both breathe a sigh of relief that this was the case. While this
may be an attempt to see things in the best light, it is possible that ME *is* best dealt with solo – if one is physically able
to do so. The nature of the illness – the sensitivity to input
from the outside world and the need to be in control –
means that it may be best endured alone. Loneliness and
hard physical challenges are weighed against waking up
every morning to a life crowded with other people's noise
and needs. Fiona believes that silence and solitude are good
housemates compared with the tensions felt and created by
others; she regards her single status as a plus, and her solitude a good context for recovery:

◆ I didn't have to cope with a partner ... it must be very
   difficult if you have to cope with a partner ... coping with
   ME is enough.

For Mike, ME was physically tough to the point where he
did not know if he could pull through on his own, but he

managed, and remains convinced that his single status helped him recover:

◆ **Being on my own allowed me to do that [pace myself] …
I didn't have to fit in with anybody else's meal patterns or
lifestyle.**

But not everyone has the opportunity to create for themselves a quiet, gentle context for recovery. Solitude is not an option for everyone, nor is it their choice. Some are too ill to live alone and others would find isolation and self-sufficiency intolerable. So how do those with partners and children cope with the demands of their loved ones and how does ME affect relationships?

Couples with ME

Of the fourteen adults, three had a husband, wife or partner who also suffered from ME. In a postal survey carried out by Action for ME, it was found that 20 per cent of severely ill people lived with family members who were similarly affected. Mothers and children were by far the most common group.

In couples, if both adults are genetically susceptible, both under stress, and both exposed to the same trigger, whether a viral agent or toxins in the environment, it is quite possible that they will both develop ME. May and her partner were stressed about a failing business when they became ill together but they report no other triggers. Mike and his wife were not ill at the same time. He was almost completely recovered when they met, but when he described his symptoms, they matched what she herself had been feeling over the previous couple of years and later she was also diagnosed with ME. Alison developed ME a year before her partner also became ill. For both of them the onset of illness coincided with vaccinations given in preparation for a trip to Tibet.

While Mike only mentions in passing that his wife has ME too, the subject is central in the interviews with both May and Alison. Yet their experiences could not be more different. As the women reflect on their feelings, it seems there is no common ground in the way they cope. For May, the experience is entirely negative. She describes a situation in which two people are ill yet unable to discuss the situation. Each suffers in silence and in solitude within the marriage. Everything is left unsaid and unexplored. May explicitly blames the acres of silence on the lack of a diagnosis. Neither she nor her husband understood what was wrong. They do not articulate the depths of exhaustion and despair which they felt, nor did they voice the need for the support each needs:

◆ It was a strain in that he didn't understand what was happening to either of us because we didn't know anything about ME … To talk to someone else who had been there, done that, would have been tremendously important.

May's husband regards her retreat into solitude as an indictment of their relationship, and interprets their illnesses as personal and emotional problems within their marriage:

◆ He felt as if I didn't love him any more which wasn't the case. It's just that I found I couldn't talk to anyone really close – either him or my mother.

So the silence which began as bafflement became entrenched as part of the way they managed and got through the illness. In complete contrast, Alison describes two people with ME living together as 'a life-saver' which brings mutual understanding, compassion and companionship:

◆ The positive part is that we know what each other is going through. And we're not alone, not only in our situation, but physically not alone. I try to imagine what it's like for somebody on their own, or somebody whose partner goes out to work every day, and I think of the long hours that must go by, and are constantly trying to do something to distract yourself, and it's too much. And knackering yourself – which doesn't really happen to us because we spend the mornings sitting in bed, do the letters, listen to the radio, do the crossword puzzle, read a book, chat, look out of the window and that's just what the mornings are like, and most of the afternoons.

She makes light of the difficulties of being shut up for seven years with a partner who is as ill as herself, dismissing the downside of entrapment with one throwaway comment:

◆ The negative side is that, well, the difficult side is that we're really on top of each other all the time, and that is what you might call a challenge.

These two relationships were already well established when ME became a third member of the household. It is a very different story when illness arrives at an earlier stage in a developing relationship when individuals are still working out the basics of how to live together. Under such circumstances the chances of a relationship surviving ME – as both of these did – is fairly minimal.

Couples: one with ME

The impact of ME on a wife, husband or partner is awful beyond description. Like any chronic illness it leads to tension, toil and heartache, but because of the uniquely unpredictable nature of ME, there is the extra element of no forward planning, no looking ahead and no tangible tomorrow. And ME is a 24/7 illness with no respite. Not surprisingly, not all marriages and relationships survive.

Everyone agreed that the strain on their partner can be even worse than the strain on themselves. As the sick partner becomes housebound or bedbound, the well one takes on the extra share of domestic responsibility, often shopping, cooking, cleaning and caring for the children, as well as going out to work. Those who take on the caring report cumulative exhaustion. There is also the wear and tear of conflicts with doctors, relatives and friends who make light of the situation, and the emotional endurance test of watching someone close to you not getting better. People with ME understand the strains imposed on their loved ones by their illness, but they are powerless to do anything about them. The other impact of ME on a close relationship – and in this respect it is probably not very different from other chronic illnesses – is that it highlights and intensifies everything. Strengths and weaknesses, tensions and bonds, are newly written in capital letters. Strain on this scale inevitably exposes the underbelly of a relationship. Established relationships are more likely to endure than more recent ones. Ray says of his relatively new relationship:

◆ I'd be quite surprised if both of us come through the other side. But it's not an impossible scenario.

Alongside the communal strain of pain and exhaustion are individual regrets, losses, difficulties and tensions. Liam regrets his loss of emotional control and bursts of bad temper which made his wife feel that she was being rejected. Alistair acknowledges the inroads into normal family life as he stopped doing all the things which, as husband and father, he used to do. He and Fraser talk about cancelled social engagements, cancelled family outings, cancelled holidays and 'just the day-to-day life that you couldn't participate in.' Janet talks about the way ME set in stone the existing incompatibility between herself and her husband, driving a final wedge between them. Ray dwells on his inability to continue to provide his girlfriend with a high standard of living. Reflecting on the difficult combination of adapting to a poorly understood illness *and* suddenly losing their financial security, he says of his partner, 'She's just struggling to take all this in.' Chloe feels guilty that her husband is deprived of a social life. The loss of friends and the inability to go out drinking represents a significant disruption to their way of living:

◆ It does affect your relationship. I feel sorry for Garry
because I can't go out for a drink. I can't drink because it
doesn't agree with me so I've not drunk for years. If we're
invited somewhere, I have to see how I feel so that affects
Garry's social life. In fact, I feel he works so hard, he
doesn't have a great social life and I feel bad about that.
You know, normally young people, you're out enjoying
yourself.

But not all husbands and partners shoulder the double
burden of work and domestic responsibility There are strik-
ing gender differences in the way people adapt to and cope
with the needs of a sick partner. A lot of the tension within
male–female relationships centres on the unfair and uneven
distribution of help and support. With a single exception,
women who need to be cared for by men have a much harder
time than men who are looked after by women. This is no
surprise since women are the carers in our society and are
already competent in that role, but it is nevertheless an indictment that even in extreme circumstances of need many
men fail to deliver and fall well short of the mark. The men
and women agree on this. The men with ME thank their
lucky stars that they have competent, compassionate wives
and they acknowledge that things would have been very different if the roles had been reversed. The women with ME
bemoan the fact that they cannot hand over the whole domestic shooting match to the men. When profoundly ill,
women still do much of the domestic orchestration. Their
men have to be programmed, chivvied and told what to do.
Denise is very stressed by the failure of her boyfriend to take

on a larger share of domestic responsibility. She argues that if he were sick, she would do everything for him, taking the initiative and allowing him space to get well. He, however, deems it a big gesture to offer her the use of his car each morning, and that's it. If she tries to talk to him he 'goes blank'. She finds his behaviour hard to forgive:

◆ A woman would do it for a man. So, yes, I have to get up early at 7am while he stays asleep. And sometimes I can't go back to sleep later. And yet I'm so tired. I'm too tired and can't rest. It's like it's gone over tiredness. Men say, 'Oh I'm not well,' and sit back for two days and the wife comes and does everything. Whereas me ... I still have to say, 'We need something for our tea tonight and the house is a mess.'

Janet talks about her husband's response to her long illness in terms that are more damning than the feeble support described by the other women. Illness brought to an end what she describes as a long ongoing struggle between the two for them for power and dominance, a battle which Janet was already losing. This marriage was an unbalanced one from the start with the 'double whammy' of him being a Scot and her being English, his conventional masculinity pitted against her gentle femininity. She felt repressed, browbeaten, forced by his coldness and silence into a relationship devoid of communication or warmth. When ME descends on such shaky foundations the whole fabric comes apart. It was as if he had finally conquered:

◆ He seemed almost to thrive on the fact that I was ill. He
remained the same. He did not want to know. He was very
shut off from it all ... he's on his path if you like and he
won't deviate to right or left. He's set in his ideas and he
won't change. He doesn't want to change. Fair enough – but
he can make me very depressed if I let him.

Janet somehow survived on her own, but seventeen years
down the line and only partly recovered, she is still angry:

◆ I get dreams now in which sometimes I'm raging at my
husband or one of my children ... the one that was so
difficult. I wake up exhausted with raging at them.

The situation is unresolved. The shell of the marriage remains
but inside it is empty. Would Janet have got better more
quickly and more fully if her husband had not turned his
back on her? Would Denise now be on the road to recovery?

The exception to the catalogue of men's inadequacies
as carers is Chloe's husband, 'a special kind of guy' who
married her when she was extremely ill, stuck by her, took
on the day-to-day domestic chores, and gave her masses of
emotional support. Here is a working-class man who comes
home after a day's work, rolls up his sleeves, and 'is doing the
hoovering and dusting and everything.' She can relax in the
knowledge that he will take care of the running of the home,
and take care of her. Not only that, he has tried hard to get
under the skin of what it is like to have ME: 'He seems to
understand ME as well as any person can understand ME.'
His compassion and hard graft make Chloe weepily guilty

that her illness has deprived him of so much. Failing to catch the irony, she describes spending the first three days of their honeymoon in bed. Her gratitude overflows:

◆ I appreciate him so much. I don't take him for granted. I appreciate everything he does for me. Not just the physical things but he's there for me. I know if I cry he's going to come and cuddle me and tell me everything is going to be all right and I will get over this. You need that support.

The men concur with the women's views and gratefully acknowledge the fact that their wives shoulder an enormous burden, effectively running the household and taking over much of what they themselves used to do as well, as well as working outside the home. Like Liam:

◆ I was fed, watered and the house was cleaned. I was buffered very significantly.

They put their recovery in part down to their wives' commitment, energy and devotion. It is a testimony to the emotional strength and stamina of Fraser's wife that she managed to cope with her sick husband, a part-time job, two young children and running the home while not displaying any frustration or anger she might have felt. Although outwardly Fraser describes her as 'coping well' he adds:

◆ I'm sure there are probably days she could have seen me far enough. Although she never came out and said it, I'm sure there were.

Alistair says much the same:

◆ She coped very well. To me she was very supportive but I
think it got her down a lot too because of the things we
couldn't do.

But there is another side to this coin; men and women
require different degrees of emotional support. In general,
the men retreat into themselves and deal with their illnesses
alone. The women are more emotionally demanding in their
wish to explore, analyse and discuss their illnesses and their
situations. They crave support and understanding, but this
may make them difficult to live with. Fraser says that while
he looked to his wife for physical help with the house and
the children, emotionally he never leant on anyone – including his wife. A brief acknowledgement of his illness was
enough:

◆ Yes, I accepted it. You know, this was my lot. It was me. It
was my turn if you like. It could have been you, him or them
over there, but it was me and that was it. I just had to get
on with it. I'm sure there were days at first when I was
feeling a bit sorry for myself, but I certainly wouldn't have
looked to anyone to pour it on. Obviously my wife was
there ... I wasn't looking for anybody to really vent my
feelings to.

This is very different from Denise whose interview is one
long cry for support.

The stoic silence of the men – and of May who manages her illness in the same way – no doubt brings its own problems. Alistair and Fraser both say that keeping their illness to themselves brings its own tensions, as silence comes to be interpreted as coldness and rejection. Alistair admits he was often bad-tempered. Liam talks with regret about the emotional coldness that was a kind of self-preservation, and his bursts of foul temper which were a response to his pain and his frustration with his symptoms. He is well aware that his inability to fulfil his share of the household chores is much less of a problem for his wife than his unpredictable moods:

◆ She could cope with the fact that I was tired, she could cope with the fact that there were certain things I couldn't do any longer … If I tried to saw a piece of wood for example it was as if I was shorted to earth. The energy went *sssssshhhhh* and I felt absurd that I had done three saws and had to go and sit down for half an hour. My wife could understand that. But the angry rejection of her, as she would perceive it, was something she couldn't accept. She couldn't come to terms with it. It was threatening and it made her feel there was something wrong with her.

Emily's story reflects that of her husband. She finds herself married to an ME-induced Jekyll and Hyde:

◆ Often two extremes of personality would exhibit themselves in an hour in that he would show complete elation and then, just like turning on a light, the other extreme would show itself – irritability, snappishness and the appearance of extreme rage.

And so, out of necessity, she adapted to solitude and, for a long time, the loss of her closest and dearest companion. Living with someone changed profoundly by ME meant drawing on immense personal resources:

He withdrew into his shell and it was a very lonely period. I had to learn over the months that I mustn't make demands and obviously I had to do a lot of things by myself. Yes, it was hard. I suppose at the beginning I resented it, I didn't understand. I remember feeling very frustrated. I remember tears, and feeling very sorry for myself. But then you realise that the man can't do anything about it, that he wasn't going to survive if there wasn't the support there, so it did feel like a dual burden in the end. Luckily, I have inner resources and there were a lot of things I could do. I didn't enter into my own pursuits wholeheartedly; it was more like a retreat. My inner resources were more like a therapy for me because all wasn't well with his life, with our life, so I got things done.

The marriage of Emily and Liam was well-established and strong when ME disrupted it. Their daughter, aged 12, was engrossed in her own life. There was a strong foundation of love, friendship and communication. But for others, ME comes too soon in a relationship bringing the threat of a split-up. Ray ponders whether his relatively new relationship will survive. The signs do not bode well since his girlfriend refuses to discuss his illness. Kirsty weeps over the break-up of her only serious relationship in eight years of illness. Chris has recently met someone he likes very much but he isn't sure that he can impose the conditions and constraints that accompany ME on someone he hardly knows. Phil describes a five-year relationship which he sustained at a time when he was still very ill – her biological clock was ticking away while for him the responsibility of caring for a child was vetoed by ME:

◆ We had five years together which came to an end three months ago because of ME basically. Last year we spent time living together to see how we could get on, and having children was a very strong need for her because her biological clock is ticking. Having children is not a strong need for me because I just envisage sleepless nights and resentment and me not being the type of father I want to be ... I don't see us getting together again and you know I've asked myself, 'Are you using ME as an excuse?', but no, I bloody am not.

For each person with ME the need – the necessity – for solitude and control is weighed in the balance against the security and support of a close, loving bond with another person. The outcome is unpredictable and uncertain.

CHAPTER 16

ME in the family: parents and siblings

> My mum understood. I had my mum. She was always there
> for me. I think as long as you've got one person on your
> side you're OK but I've heard terrible stories where people
> have had nobody, not even their family, and that must be
> horrendous.
> CHLOE

Young people with ME do their best to maintain an equilibrium within the family which contains and cares for them, but they are aware of the tensions which ripple through the household as a result of their illness and so gratitude and frustration live uneasily side by side. Trapped under the same roof as their parents and siblings, it is inevitable that they pick up on any bad vibes. It is significant that Jessie uses the word 'feel' rather than 'know' to describe how she is tuned in to the feelings of her family; the tension is felt in the air, something so tangible that it bypasses thought:

◆ I feel how it affects the rest of the family. I kind of feel
guilty for it sometimes. It's better now than it was, but the
family was much more stressed out than it would have been
otherwise, and it showed on everyone.

She uses the word 'stressed out' over and over as she talks about her illness and its impact on her parents and siblings. And so not for these young people the careless, throwaway attitudes of their teenage peers who treat their parents as doormats or the providers of hotel accommodation. Young people with ME remain vigilant, protective and overcaring as they monitor the tensions and unhappiness which they themselves cause.

There is also conflict between parents as they disagree about the best way to manage their child's illness. Usually the conflict centres around a mother who believes and accepts the severity of her child's illness pitted against a father who cajoles and bullies his offspring into trying harder. Sometimes fathers simply bury their heads in the sand. Ill children hear the whispered conversations, the raised voices, the outbursts of despair and they live in the angry silences.

Parents and their children

Lizzie describes the mother–child relationship as 'a really difficult dynamic.' It is a tough one, fraught with problems and hazards. How do mothers and their growing children negotiate such an emotionally charged situation? Those in their late teens and early twenties would, if ME had not happened, have flown the nest and be enjoying their first taste of freedom and independence. Instead, they crawl back wounded or, like Josh and David and Rachel, are too ill to leave home at all.

Young people have a lot to say about the conflicting emotions of needing to be cared for like a child, yet wishing for the freedom of an adult. They struggle with difficult feelings at a time when they are already vulnerable because they are so ill. All talk about their painful yet necessary dependence on their parents, and about the lack of control over their own lives. They talk about containing warring emotions of gratitude and resentment, dependence and restlessness, childlike needs and grown-up longings. Jessie says of her mother:

◆ I totally rely on her. I used to find that hard. I used to feel kind of trapped and stuff. I still do.

While parents try to create a separate living space and some sort of independence for their children, both parties know it is a sham. The young people are conscious that their space is within their parents' space and that they have little control over the family timetable and agenda. Somewhere along the line many young people realise that it is less draining to endure the situation than to put up a futile battle against it. Josh says that he has lashed out at his mother only a couple of times. On one occasion they had been discussing the possibility of his trying to live with support in his own flat:

◆ My mum said she would pitch in and help with food and so on and I said, 'That's the whole point. I don't want you to "pitch in". I'm sick of being babied. Sick of not being responsible for myself. I want to look after myself. I don't want you to look after me.'

Young people go home to be cared for only as a last resort. It is the final option when they cannot look after themselves any longer. Despite being extremely ill for ten years, Chris hung on in a shared flat, determined to keep a toehold on independence. Although it would have been easier at a physical level to have someone else do the shopping, prepare the meals and run him around, the sacrifice in terms of his dignity and self-esteem was too great:

◆ I don't think I could. People have said to me, 'Why don't you go home to your parents?', but it would be such a backward step. I just don't think psychologically I could cope. I couldn't cope with that. I've lost so many other things, you know.

Going home represents a loss of control, a shift of role and a loss of status. It means retracing their footsteps to a place they have left behind. Chris says for him it would have been too great a sacrifice. Jessie says the same. Returning home is the equivalent of giving up, but one year into her university course when she finally achieved freedom both from the worst of her symptoms and from the parental home, she had to do it. She describes the move as 'horrible':

◆ I didn't want to have to move home. It felt like I just gave up. I was just giving in and going backwards, you know, like it was crashing round my ears. It's still pretty depressing having to move back home and give up. I felt like I was losing my independence and, yeah, losing my freedom. I loved the fact that I could just do what I wanted and nobody knew what I was doing.

Going home, staying at home, being cared for like a child, is only the best of a very bad bunch of options. It is never a positive choice.

Mothers and sons; mothers and daughters

Mothers are described as pivotal figures in the ME scenario. They are at the epicentre of both the caring and of the domestic tensions. They are courageous figures often struggling under painful emotional burdens. Mum is described as the central and most significant person by the children and young people with ME. She is the one who does not question the reality of her child's illness and the one who understands. Kirsty describes her mum as her 'best friend'. Jessie says her mother is 'the only one who really understands'. Josh describes his mum as 'a good mother'. They are also the key players in the battles with the medical and educational establishments, trying to protect their children from inappropriate treatment and care.

But mothers walk an emotional tightrope between the needs of a sick child and those of a young adult. On the one hand, young people lean on their mothers who are often, by default, their daily and only companions; on the other hand, growing children want to be free of this childlike dependence and yearn to wriggle out from the umbrella of support which their mothers provide. Mum ends up as piggy-in-the-middle. With the best will in the world, it is hard to get the relationship right. While young people acknowledge the selfless support which their mothers give, and express their gratitude, they also talk about more ambivalent feelings, wanting more freedom and independence than their mothers perhaps provide. I interviewed Kirsty a couple of days after she had returned from a short trip away. In her absence, her mother had redecorated her room. It was meant to be a surprise:

◆ I went away last week and when I came back my mum had actually painted my bedroom. My bedroom is like, you know, my zone, and as much as it was a good intention, I actually felt quite gutted. I thought: 'This is like I'm not in control of my own life. I don't have somewhere that's mine.' I know it was with good intentions, but the colour is kind of fluorescent! She painted it lime green. When I opened my bedroom door I just felt a big lump. I felt this was done with the best of intentions, but it was like, 'No!' I felt I needed control … no, not control … the space. I don't have the energy to go out so space is important to me. I didn't realise how important it was until Friday. I just felt the floor was taken from beneath me when this happened.

Kirsty is, after all, 22 years old. She describes her room as her only private space so an intrusion with a paintbrush felt very bad indeed. So too does the invasion of her privacy every morning by her young nephew:

◆ He comes round at seven in the morning. He's learnt to open my door and come into my bedroom and it's almost an encroachment of my space.

Why on earth does she say 'almost'? Jessie feels similarly trapped by her illness as she copes with feelings of resentment, at once more becoming needy and dependent on her mother after the freedom of a year away at university:

◆ It's hard. I totally rely on her. I used to find that hard. I used to feel kind of trapped. I still do.

Most mothers recognise the difficulties of both caring for a young person with ME who may be in their teens or twenties, and the need to give them a bit of space and privacy. But it is hard to provide what is after all only an illusion of independence. Mothers don't need to be accused by doctors and teachers of being overprotective because they already accuse themselves. Marilyn was told by several doctors that she was 'a neurotic mother' keeping her son housebound and ill. But is this an overprotective mother talking?

◆ We used to run a business from home so I got myself a part-time job to give David some space to develop as a person. I didn't feel he could develop with me always there. So he had space in the house. I love David so much. I'd just do anything for him. But I will always stand back and let him be his own person. I'm always just there for him when he's needing anything.

Another mother phoned to say that although their son is only 25 per cent better, they are making arrangements for him to leave the family home:

◆ It is necessary for him and necessary for us. We can't go on any longer like this.

Rachel thinks that her mother's full-time job has helped her cope with her illness by giving her a life outside the sickroom. Acknowledging both the problems of a mother and child cooped up together as well as the horror of the severity of her illness, she says:

◆ One person I know who also has it, her mum doesn't work.
  She looks after her all the time. Her mum is on the point of
  cracking up, she really is, because there's no getting away
  from it … my parents have coped very well considering that
  they nearly lost me.

One problem is that all outward markers of time passing,
and of children maturing, are missing. There are no rites of
passage: no first night at the pub, no first all-night party,
no driving test. Maybe no boyfriend or girlfriend. The years
pass, children remain at home, and it is not always possible
to see clearly enough that they are maturing and changing.
The tussles and flare-ups of normal adolescence, the nego-
tiations for more time or territory, the full-on fights are all
absent. Children do not have the energy to quarrel with their
mothers, nor do they have much to quarrel about.

Unfortunately, mothers can also create feelings of guilt as
tensions grow in previously healthy households, and as they
try – and fail – to hide their own anguish. There is no blame
to be apportioned here, only understanding. Young people
are made particularly observant by a chronic illness which
forces them to play a passive, watching role. Ruby, age 14,
expresses her own grief and anger at the anguish her mother
has been through after being diagnosed with Munchhausen's syndrome by proxy. Jessie says:

◆ I hate seeing the effect it has on Mum, you know.
  Obviously, it really upsets her. I do feel guilty for the stress
  that it's put on her, and the rest of the family. You know it's
  terrible seeing your mum totally stressed out when you

know you're the cause. I can't even do anything for myself most of the time. I was in bed. Not exactly bedbound, but I was in bed. But, yeah, I was totally dependent on her. I wasn't doing much at all. Now, when I'm home, she cooks and she washes and stuff. She's a very caring mother anyway, but ...

And what is left unsaid is that she wishes more than words can say that she does not need to be cared for by her mother. It is no longer appropriate – but it has to be.

Then there is the problem of overidentification with a sick child. When maternal emotions are running high it is hard not to be sucked deeply into the illness, almost living the ME with the child rather than remaining cool, detached yet caring. In these circumstances, the emotional situation becomes confusing, tortuous and overheated. Lizzie, talking about her mother, sympathetically describes the daily tension:

She very much related to me. I think it was very confusing for her because she maybe overidentified. It's a very difficult thing anyway because we were the complete thing in her life – three children. I mean, it's easy for me to say – I haven't got children – but it was difficult for her to separate and say, 'This is Lizzie's illness. This is Lizzie's thing to work through.' And I think she felt guilty. You know, then I would feel guilty that she was feeling guilty. And I'd feel grumpy and frustrated as a teenager that she was clinging, and too worrying.

My own emotions as the mother of an ill son whom I love, admire and respect have at times been more than I could bear. Sometimes I have walked the pavements in tears of rage and despair at his pain, patience, endurance and loss. Probably other mothers have done the same. While mothers do not want to further burden their children with their anguish, there is a limit to their own emotional endurance. Sometimes an upbeat voice sounds horribly false and a smile becomes a grimace. Wise children know what mothers are going through, and all of them acknowledge their suffering.

I hope that I have not been too hard on mothers in these pages. They are in an impossible situation, trying to do an impossible job. It is terribly difficult to achieve a balance between providing and caring on the one hand, and not being overprotective or overinvolved on the other. If I have been critical, it is because I am the mother of a 19-year-old son with ME, and I daily feel my own inadequacies.

Fathers and sons; fathers and daughters

In general, fathers feature little in the interviews. They are remarkable mainly for their absence – literally, in the case of Marilyn and David:

◆ I used to get up at least twice in the night to make his meals and I had to get up in the morning and go to work. There was one occasion when I just couldn't get out of bed so I asked him to ask his dad. His dad turned round and said, 'Get it yourself.' From then on, I never asked John to do anything for David, and David never asked him either.

John walked out on his wife and son five years into David's illness. Marilyn blames the breakdown of her marriage on her husband's inability to come to terms with his son having ME.

If they do stay the course, fathers seem to play a more distant role, hardly appearing in the interviews. One reason is that they are away at work all day and so do not witness the hourly struggles because they are not the ones providing the daily care. But it is more than this: the young people say that while their mothers unconditionally accept the awfulness of their illness, their fathers are not so sure. Fathers seem more reluctant, or less able, to come to terms with the reality of ME; they are reported as more dismissive, less communicative, more ready to urge their ill son or daughter to try harder, more eager to try to get them back to school. Kirsty says:

◆ I think the only person that really knows me when I'm ill is my mum. Even, I suppose, my dad, he'll come home from work at night-time and think: 'Well, she looks OK now.' But my mum is with me most of the time so she's the only person that really sees me all the time.

Before Jessie was first diagnosed as suffering from ME, and when neither parent knew much about it, both tried to push her into doing more than she could:

◆ Everyone was trying to get me to go to school all the time when I didn't feel well and we'd have battles every day. You know, them trying to force me to go to school and me not feeling well enough. They just wanted me at school.

Later, when it was clear that her illness was severe and entrenched, her mother accepted the situation and let her be while her father, like most of the fathers described in the transcripts, never really came to terms with her suffering:

◆ My mum's great. She's very sympathetic, very. She looks after me and she's great. My dad has always been a step back from it. He's always been out at work and he's not the most sympathetic person anyway. I mean I don't get any sympathy from him. Not that I particularly want sympathy, but he's not the most understanding person. Yeah, we've had our run-ins.

My personal experience conflicts with the majority view of fathers as background players. Perhaps my experience reflects the fact that I too am ill, but without my husband's support I wonder how my son and I would have survived. For almost four years, cut off physically and socially in a tiny, socially ingrown Scottish village, he has been the packhorse from the supermarket, the chauffeur, the calm charger into battles with doctors, our link to the outside word, our lifeline, and a bottomless pit of support. My son says of him, 'I think fathers can sometimes cope better than mothers.'

And the very distance which fathers place between themselves and their sick children can be an advantage. Because they return from the world of work to the sick world, because they are not closeted all day with a sick child, and because they are not the ones to see and hear their children's most painful emotions, they can bring to the situation a greater sense of ordinariness and calm. Prosaic interactions may be exactly what are needed.

Brothers and sisters

ME, like other severe illnesses, changes and reshapes the entire family. It's as if the normal family snapshot of two of three children lined up with smiles in front of their parents is completely re-arranged. Now the sick child is right in the middle, dominating the photo – the other children have faded into the background. The parents reach out towards the child in the middle. A sick child, especially one with a chronic illness, creates anxiety and tensions which reverberate around the whole family. Despite the best attempts to treat a young person with ME as 'normally' as possible, that normality is a necessary charade and a thinly-veiled illusion. In reality, ME dominates and disrupts family life, often deeply. It is widely accepted that chronic illness in the family affects all the children, not just the one who is sick. A study of the brothers and sisters of child cancer sufferers[1] shows that six months after diagnosis, a quarter of siblings were still showing emotional and behavioural problems. They reported feeling resentment at the lack of attention they received, and guilty that they felt resentment. These are complex emotions for children to deal with. The young people I interviewed talked about the effect of their illness on their siblings, especially young brothers and sisters who found themselves displaced as the focus of their parents' attention. Inevitably, there is resentment from the healthy children, and guilt felt by the sick one. Jessie talks about the way her long illness robbed her younger sister of her prominent place in the family, pushing her to one side as their mother concentrated her physical and emotional resources on the older, ill sister.

◆ The stress showed on everyone. On Katy, my little sister.
Katy is a very attention-seeking child anyway so it just made
it worse – the fact that I did need so much attention from
my mum, and she wanted the attention for herself.

One manifestation of deep-seated resentment on the part of
siblings is to underplay the extent of their brother's or sister's
suffering. This seems to be what is happening in Kirsty's
family as her siblings downplay her plight, refuse to accept
the severity of her symptoms, and fail to offer help and
support. Kirsty belongs to a big family. When she became
too ill to take care of herself, she returned home to be looked
after by her mother, but not before trying to manage on her
own. She picked up resentment from her siblings, even from
the two older sisters who were married and had left home.
This response may reflect their own needs and emotions more
than the needs of the sick member of the household. Kirsty's
sisters' refusal to accept or discuss her situation seems to stem
from their perception of her as the favoured one, the over-
protected one, still at home being cared for by Mum. The
reality is that Kirsty remains very ill after nine years of illness,
largely confined to the house, and still in need of considerable
support. Although 22 years old, Kirsty has to accept that
in terms of her physical needs, she remains a child. Her
two older sisters don't accept this, regarding her continuing
presence there as a choice rather than a necessity. Instead of
sympathy there is a stony silence on the topic of ME:

◆ My sisters come round and they don't even say, 'How are
you?' or anything like that, but I've learned to live with it

and it's OK. I get used to it but you think it's funny the way
they must perceive me.

She describes how jealousy and resentment warp reality to
the point where they seem to believe that it is more desirable
to be sick and housebound than to be well and independent:

◆ I think maybe, in a way, why they haven't accepted the ME,
is they're jealous of the relationship between my mum and I.
I don't know but they say, 'Gosh, you're lucky to not have
to go out and work.' But it's not. I'd give my back teeth to
go out to work. If I'm going out, I'm going out with my mum,
whereas my sisters think, 'How come she is going out with
my mum and we can't.' It's silly, it's almost like being
childlike again and yet my sisters are 28 and 27, and they've
got their own families now. For a while my sister's boyfriend
and my sister they were saying, 'Yeah, you could get a
place. There's a nice house for you. You should get a place
of your own.' Financially, where do I get this, you know? It
would be lovely to have my own place and one day I will,
but at the moment there's really no other option.

In contrast, Kirsty's brother was at home when she 'hit rock
bottom' and so witnessed her day-by-day decline into profound disability. He does believe in ME, and offers support
the best way he can by coming up with possible explanations for her illness and practical solutions.

◆ When I was really sort of severely paralysed he said, 'You
know, I've heard that smoking hash cures ME and helps. I

could get you some if you wanted.' I thought, although, yes it was illegal, it showed that he had thought about it and was willing to do something to help me and I was really quite touched at that and I thought: 'Gosh, that says a lot for him.' And even now – he's an agricultural student – and he's saying, 'You know, I think water maybe causes ME', and he's coming up with these things, so he's always sort of still thinking about me which is really nice.

Kirsty's quiet acceptance of the inadequacy of her sisters' response, and her gratitude for the comfort she gets from her brother is both moving and disquieting. She is forgiving, and generous in her acceptance of their inadequacies:

⬦ Even after eight years, they don't really understand. It's not their fault at all but they don't really understand. Maybe they just want a normal sister. I don't know.

The loss of the chance to have a family

For three women – Alison, Chloe and Dawn – ME means the loss of a chance to have a family because they are too ill to contemplate caring for a child. Personally, I know of two others. Time passes, they do not get better, and eventually it is too late.

Alison met Peter when she was 38, hoping to start a family soon. Seven years have passed, they remain ill, and Alison's biological clock registers that it is now too late. Struggling at first to embark on this personal subject, she nevertheless talks about her situation positively, not in terms of loss. Perhaps her acceptance is a matter of emotional self-preservation, perhaps a way of coming to terms with the inevitable reality, or perhaps a reflection of her Buddhist philosophy:

◆ One of the things that ... it's just that ... we don't have children. Not having children could be an enormous grief to me but, my God, I'm so glad I don't have children, with this. I mean how could I, how could we possibly ... Peter and I only got together when I was 38. If I'd said, 'Right, we've got to have a child now because it will be too late.' I would have had a child aged four when I got this. Well, it would have been taken away. I wouldn't ... Peter and I couldn't have brought it up. You know, so it's got to be a course of rejoicing that I haven't got a child. I've got to be positively happy, I mean I am positively happy that I haven't got a child who has been taken away from me, you know.

We ended there. Neither of us had the heart to talk about anything else.

This is an emotionally raw subject. It is testimony to the women's wish to leave nothing about this illness unvoiced that they are willing to open their hearts on such a deeply personal issue. In one of the support groups in California, Dawn bowed her head when she said, 'I never had kids.' The other women acknowledged her loss by remaining silent, and bowing their heads with her. And Chloe's tears are more powerful than the words she used to describe her desolation at the prospect of remaining childless:

◆ I am 32 now, so I would absolutely love to have a baby. That's something that has had to be put on hold. And then I'm thinking about the future, you know: 'Am I going to have a baby?' That's something I've always wanted. So that's quite hard ... I feel my future has been taken away. Most people my age would be planning to have a baby. I can plan nothing, and that's really upsetting.

At this point, Chloe broke down and wept. Once again it felt right to end the interview.

Caring for the carers?

The carers are heroic and selfless as they cope with sick family members, battle with doctors and teachers, stand between their ill children and threats of inappropriate treatment, and all the while try to keep their own lives ticking over. How much they shoulder; and for how long. Yet none of those I interviewed received due recognition, acknowledgement and kindness from their families nor the kind of support and sympathy that would have made their lives a bit more tolerable. What they report is intolerance, hardness and an isolating silence from their own relatives and in-laws – the very people who should have been there for them.

Coping with a loved one who is ill is a lonely business, but that loneliness is intensified when relatives pretend that nothing much is wrong and imply that the carer is laying it on with a trowel when they describe the inroads made by ME on the whole family. Silence magnifies the isolation imposed by illness and reinforces the sense of difference that is already keenly felt. Emily talked a lot about having to find and draw on her own inner resources because basically she was alone as she watched and dealt with her husband's illness. She says:

◆ It was frustrating. Especially in the early days when ME wasn't recognised. It was very difficult explaining to people. A lot of my time was spent making excuses for him – why he could not do that – and withdrawing into myself because from people who were close, especially relatives, one got all sorts of gratuitous advice and platitudes. Like, 'Why doesn't he take a holiday?' And 'Oh well, go and take yourselves off for a fortnight to the sun', as if a day in a deckchair was all that was needed. And you would try to explain, but that's all you would get, so you didn't bother explaining. They were the ones who came up with the explanation, 'Do you think, dear, it might just be in the mind'.

Emily did what others did. She stopped trying, stopped explaining, and more or less stopped talking to relatives who refused to listen. One of the key problems with ME, as the carers found, was that relatives were willing to listen to their bulletins of a total lack of progress for a short time but then they switched off. Their patience was exhausted. They did not understand ME and did not seem willing to try to understand what their siblings and children were actually dealing with:

◆ I think I put forward my point of view, and initially it was sympathetically received, but within three or four months there was this assumption that he was better now. And you

221

explain again for another three or four months. By the time you get to a year you just give the response, 'Yes, we're coping.' I withdrew. I cut myself off. I just didn't expose myself to it.

Ann, the single mother who was accused of Munchhausen's syndrome by proxy, literally wrung her hands as she spoke of the refusal of her family to believe her account of what was happening. Incredibly, neither her parents nor her siblings believed in Ruby's illness. She describes a time when she had to leave Ruby with her parents for a couple of days while she attended a conference, and with the unpredictable fickleness typical of ME, Ruby was in a relatively good phase and probably did what everyone with ME does – she wound herself up so that she *would* cope with a different environment and a different routine. Later she would collapse – but that of course was at home:

◆ They didn't see anything really wrong with her. I was so upset because when I went to pick her up I got taken aside and my mother said to me, 'You know, Dad and I have been thinking, and we don't think there's anything the matter with her. We think it's school phobia. We're convinced it's school phobia.' We got into an acrimonious argument about it because she was emphatic there was nothing wrong. You see, my mother was a nurse.

So the grandmother who was a nurse and who saw Ruby for a few days now and again knew better than the mother who lived with and cared for her seriously ill child. It is not an unusual story. But the lack of a medical qualification doesn't bar others from dishing out their psychobabble or, by adopting a silence in which they never even ask about the person who is ill, making it obvious that they don't believe in ME. Nelson, who has wider shoulders than most people, talked with obvious sadness about the way his parents and siblings quickly turned their backs on him. They knew better than he did what was wrong in the family, and with his son Josh, and with his wife who also suffered from a chronic illness. The messages relayed back – and the messages were always veiled and implied rather than explicit – was either that Nelson and his wife were exaggerating, or that the whole family was dysfunctional. It was something the psychiatrists should be dealing with:

◆ My wife's family have been pretty good. They haven't pretended to understand but they have been willing to take things on trust. If you say you're ill, you're ill. If you say Josh is ill, he's ill, however implausible the situation got like some B horror movie. They didn't question sanity. I wish I could say the same for mine. I don't know if this is a typical pattern of husbands' family distrust because it is true that my family had a somewhat strained relationship with my wife before this happened, but I was truly amazed that my family basically could not bring itself to believe in ME. My mother has finally come round and acknowledges what we have been through. But the others not. Of course, there was nothing as simple as outright denial, but nevertheless my brother and sister have never taken on board the fact that two out of four of my family have suffered a seriously

debilitating illness over a period of a dozen years. Their
attitude has had the effect of estrangement. It has been
more hurtful than I think I have been prepared to admit. In
a way it's the feature of the affair what I least understand.

For Ann and Nelson, years of coping with loved ones in a
climate of disbelief from the medical profession, from the
education establishments, and even from their own families,
has resulted in a deterioration in their own health. Ann is
very depressed and stretched to breaking point. Nelson is
suffering from a stress-related illness himself. But it is the
attitudes of others, even more than the illness itself, which
has most contributed to their distress and their isolation, as
Nelson says:

◆ The upshot of these interactions with the outside world's
   attitude to ME is isolation. By comparison, dealing with the
   illness is less of the equation than one would expect.

In the balance against family attitudes like these, one weighs
the fact that at one point Josh's GP warned Nelson and his
wife that their son was so weak and fragile that he was in
danger of dying.

CHAPTER 17

Seeking support

There is a brotherhood of those who bear
the mark of pain.
ALBERT SCHWEITZER[1]

The men, women and young people with ME turned in different directions for support to help them through the difficult years. For the men able to work there was solace in the routine and familiarity of the workplace, and sanity in the banter of their colleagues – not for them the ME ghetto with its talk of illness. But others, whose lives are dominated by the presence of ME, needed sympathy, and needed to exchange progress reports with others in the same boat. They talk about illness because their illness engulfs them. In most of the narratives there is some support, though often minimal and not always from expected sources. Support is the local ME group; the husband or sister who understands; the dog or cat who stays at the bedside; the loyal friend on the end of the phone; e-mail contact and the internet chat room; cards and letters; a newsletter mailed by a national association. It is the ME grapevine. The security of the ME ghetto. Very few manage to go it alone. From the severely ill and housebound comes a cry for more practical help and moral support. Either it is not there – or they are too ill to access it.

What follows is a distillation of how people found, or failed to find, the sympathy and support which was right for them.

National support groups

The two long-established national organisations for people with ME in the UK, the ME Association and Action for ME, offer helplines, penfriend schemes, meetings up and down the country, information about local and special interest groups, research reports, and regular newsletters and magazines. Yet in my sample, most people found membership of these organisations unhelpful and unappealing. Alison, typical of many, gave the newsletters a try in the early stages of her illness but soon abandoned them because she found them depressing:

◆ I've joined all of them I think. And I've given them all up. I belonged to Action for ME for a couple of years and the ME Association for a couple of years and their magazines were so full of ghastly stories that Peter wouldn't even read them and I would read them and take a week to recover. So I gave up my subscriptions for those – I didn't want to know. They never seemed to report people getting better after a couple of years or something.

Many sympathised with this point of view, saying that ploughing through depressing and repetitive stories of illness, and reading about unproven, anecdotal accounts of remedies and therapies was neither helpful nor encouraging. Instead, they preferred to take a short walk or talk to a friend. They wanted to be distracted from ME if there was nothing definite or positive to be said about it. Most people described the national magazines as 'depressing'.

I became so distressed with the national magazines in the early stages of my illness that my son would intercept them and put them in the bin. But that was sixteen years ago. Since then, the national associations have grown up and moved on. They produce more professional, informative, balanced publications. And my expectations are different. Whereas at one time I scanned the pages for cures, treatments, stories of people who had recovered, now I accept that my illness is chronic and that there are no such rainbows. I use the magazine to keep abreast of developments in the research field, and to keep in touch with the experiences of others.

Local support groups

Some swear by local groups while others give them a wide berth because within their closed circles the ME label is written in capital letters. Local support groups come in different shapes and sizes but still they do not fit everyone. For some they are a lifeline; for others depressing and self-absorbed. One of the main criticisms is that they can become cliques, run for years and years by the same people with chronic ME until the group becomes stale and tedious. The other complaint is that local support groups can degenerate into chatty, gossipy sessions dominated by individual case histories when what is needed is information, action, invited speakers who have something useful to say, and talks by sympathetic doctors and alternative practitioners who have something practical to offer. In my sample, the majority of people reported that either they had not bothered to contact a local support group because they had been warned what to expect, or had attended one or two meetings only to find them dreary, depressing and unhelpful.

At first glance there seems to be the expected gender differences in the wish to attend support groups or to make contact with others with ME. Most of the men avoid the entire ME circuit, instead sticking to long-standing friends and colleagues who knew them before they became ill. The last thing Fraser, Liam and Alistair wanted was a formal or informal group organised around ME. But while more women than men contacted and attended support groups, the differences go beyond gender. The men, as a group, were not as sick, and therefore not as isolated as the women and so were able to keep going in the workplace. The women turned to others with ME in formal and informal contexts because they were cut off from the workplace and had lost their social life. In fact, the women who were less severely ill said much the same as the men – that they preferred to seek support outside the ME network, like Fiona who chose to do voluntary work with disabled people when depression threatened to overwhelm her one year into ME. On the other hand, the men who were very ill, unable to work, and housebound, did seek others with ME, just like the women.

During the fifteen-year course of my illness I have encountered the worst and the best of support groups. I remember a day in the first year of my relapse: a day of despair and tears. I rang someone listed in the local ME group. I was very ill and easily tired. The woman on the end of the helpline asked me briefly about my illness and then chatted for an hour about her own case history. It was so bad I had to put the phone down on the bed and bury my head in the pillow. She did not appear to notice the lack of response or the silence because the voice just droned on. That was my first and last contact with the group. Instead, I discovered effective support through the local MEIT (ME Information Technology) group run by a few dedicated people who trawled the internet for new developments in research and treatment and then regularly sent out useful, informative and encouraging packs of material. E-mail was easier than the telephone because one could skip the social niceties, and a cry for help always got a quick and helpful response. This was exactly what I needed.

Cognitive-behavioural classes in California

Two years on from this experience, and newly arrived in California, I went along to the first of a series of self-help classes which, fortuitously, were just starting in my neighbourhood. Bruce Campbell, the group leader, developed the concepts and wrote the manual for the classes[2] as he recovered from his own experience of ME, drawing on his considerable knowledge of cognitive-behavioural programs, taking the best from this contentious method of treating ME and abandoning the rest. A full account of Bruce's own recovery can be found on the CFIDS self-help website (*see* Resources, page 326). In a recent communication he writes:

◆ I would like to stress the interactive nature of the
relationship between the development of our course and
my recovery, and also the many sources used to create the
program. I started the courses with the assumption that
together a group of patients could figure out how to
improve. In structuring the course, I made use of elements
from Kate Lorig's self-help programs from Stanford, David
Spiegel's breast cancer support groups, the work of Alicia
Deale applying Cognitive Behavioral Therapy in individual
therapy with CFS patients, and twelve-step programs. In the
first of several sets of groups, I tried to discover what was
helpful, using these other sources, the experiences of group
members and my own experience. My conclusions were
then expressed as the principles of the course, which I then
used as the standards to guide my own recovery.

This was a very different affair from the claustrophobic,
chatty, anecdotal evenings I had attended – and quickly
abandoned – in Edinburgh. The self-help programme was
based on the three key concepts of self-help, living within
one's limits, and finding effective coping strategies. Each
class ran for an hour and a half, dealt with a theme such as
Managing Stress, and was split into three manageable half-
hour sessions. Bruce kept tight reins on the proceedings,
began punctually, ended on time, and guided us back if we
strayed off course. Cast in stone was the rule that within
each half-hour session, everyone had the opportunity to talk
for a maximum of five minutes without interruption; that
way no one hogged the limelight, no one wore everyone else
out with lengthy personal sagas, and diffident members

were given the opportunity to speak. We were encouraged to be positive and creative in the way we talked about illness, and to offer tools and techniques for management rather than degenerating into self-pity. Usually we operated within the constraints Bruce set, and most of the time it worked extremely well, but occasionally when we hit an emotive note, or when someone became upset, then maybe he should have sat back, abandoned his tight schedule and let the group talk itself out.

But the cognitive-behavioural approach was not always appropriate, nor was it right for everyone. It assumed (correctly for people who were completely out of tune with their bodies or who totally denied the reality of their illness) that everyone would benefit from explicit objectives and weekly targets. But no one should ever have told Ruth what to do. She *knew* instinctively what her body could take, and how much mental and emotional energy she dared to expend. She had been ill with fibromyalgia for eighteen years and was perfectly in tune with the ebb and flow of her energy levels. Out of necessity she listened for signals to push forward a bit or to put the brakes on. Ruth finally agreed to set a target of walking each day as far as the communal dining room. But this fixed goal made her much worse. Trying to walk a set distance at a set time each day, irrespective of how she felt, resulted in a dramatic increase of symptoms. She gave a tearful reporting back at the following class, propped up on a dozen cushions, pale as a ghost and unable to move even her fingers without intense pain:

◆ I forced it through. I walked to the dining hall and stayed to dinner because I was trapped. I could not get back.

This was one of very few negative experiences in three months of meetings. At the first session everyone introduced themselves and immediately there was a strong sense of sharing and a bonding. We ceased to be a collection of individuals and became a committed group whose members cared deeply about one another, wanting to help in positive ways. The bonds which were created in that first session lasted throughout and between the classes – so strong in fact that two potential new members felt unable to penetrate our tightly-knit circle and did not return. In this support group, members were an inspiration to one another, giving those who were flagging renewed zest to carry on. Back in the UK, I miss the self-help classes and the wise and wonderful people who for a while were a significant part of my life.

The best support groups should be like this. It should feel good to enter the room, see the warm welcoming faces, and sense the shared emotions and experiences. In such contexts, people with ME can relax into a space and time set aside for helping one another in an atmosphere which is non-judgemental and tolerant, so that they feel free to be themselves. This is a setting in which people nod their heads or reach out a hand, because they truly understand what is being recounted. In our group, occasionally we wept because someone was describing so accurately and exactly what we ourselves had experienced. Their reality was our reality. By making their experiences explicit, they were given validity.

Recent studies of the powerful impact of effective support

groups reinforce my own experience in California. Women with breast cancer who participated in therapeutic support groups lived an average of eighteen months longer than those who only received medical care.[3] Dr Spiegel, interviewed in *Arthritis Today*, said that he found the result surprising because while he had expected that the women would be helped emotionally, he did not expect a significant difference in the length of time they survived with cancer.[4] Surprised by the interrelationship of emotional and physical well-being, he was forced to conclude that the intense social support the women received helped them feel less overwhelmed and more in control of their disease.

Retreat to the ME ghetto

The word retreat is a military term which means getting the hell out of somewhere bad. In the context of ME, retreat means backing off from the pressures of the normal world and from the stress of relating to healthy people. It is moving to a quieter back road where energy is not consumed in pointless explanation and argument. It is perhaps the end of a long road, not a choice or an option, but simply where, by default, one winds up.

Sometimes it becomes too painful to struggle on in the world of the well. To outsiders, this may seem like a cop out, but a retreat into the ME ghetto can be a positive move, offering a safe haven in which to come to terms with a difficult illness and a different way of living. Amongst others who are similarly stranded and sick, one does not feel dysfunctional or a freak. In a society where the attitudes of the healthy induce feelings of guilt and powerlessness, for many it makes a lot of sense to turn instead to others in the same boat. Within the ME ghetto, individuals choose friends and allies as they would in any other social context.

Perhaps the main attraction of the ME ghetto is that within it one can redefine normality. Alison's retreat has a double meaning. It is both a physical removal from 'real life', stranded on the fifth floor of a tenement building with baskets of food hoisted up on a rope, and a psychological tool for survival. When she says, 'Yes. We are normal. The rest of the world isn't', she knows that this is both true and untrue. It is a game she plays to get through the empty days. It is also a genuine normality because for seven years there has been no other reality and with time comes necessary and inevitable adaptation. ME is an imposed, open-ended retreat, bringing all kinds of hardship, yet Alison embraces and accepts it, comparing herself positively to others who enter into a retreat for religious or spiritual reasons:

◆ The highest form of life is being a retreatant. The people whom I have most esteem are people who have put themselves through a retreat, a three or four year retreat, and some of them have done it twice. That is to be cut off in a way that I can't imagine … This is a hotel retreat. We've got luxury.

Like Ruth, Alison's acceptance of enforced solitude has its roots in a deep spirituality. Her stoicism and ability to deal with frustration are breathtaking. She has been too ill to play the piano for seven years. She bought a viol because it is a lighter, more delicate instrument, but has not progressed far. When she manages to get to a group class, she sits at the back, hopelessly behind the others, knowing she will pay the price for just being there, in the noisy atmosphere of tuning strings and talking and laughter, and that she will be shattered for days afterwards.

Chloe too knows that her redefinition of normal is a safety net, a strategy, something to keep her sane, and a way of dealing with her illness, but unlike Alison's forbearance she struggles against it. Over and again in her interview she says that her new normality is imposed and unwanted:

◆ It's not normal. I do not live a normal life. I mean, it's normal for me now. That's my life. I try to enjoy what I can ... but I just really want to be fully fit and able to work and have a social life just like a normal person. I was very sociable whereas now I suppose you would call me very unsociable but that's not due to choice. I would love to go out.

But her friends fail to understand that she cannot stay out late, or drink, or join in all the activities she once enjoyed, so Chloe too turns inwards to the ME ghetto to seek people who have no preconceived expectations of her. She has finally turned her back on her 'normal' friends and found a yoga class for disabled people:

◆ I find that fantastic. It's a class full of MS and ME people and I find that great because we all understand one another and the instructor actually has MS himself so you get a lot of strength from that group. There's a lot of breathing techniques and you just do exactly what you want. If you're having a bad day, you just do a little. It's been a godsend.

She has also found support among others with ME:

◆ For all we don't see each other a lot, we're on the phone which is nice, and you know exactly how they are feeling, and they know how you are feeling because they are going through it themselves.

The leitmotif in the many accounts of people seeking support within the ME ghetto is that only there do people understand. There is no need to explain. There is acceptance and validation.

Another reason for retreating to the ME ghetto is that social interaction with people who do not have ME is too draining. The invisible cognitive disabilities which make concentrating on conversation so difficult and exhausting go unrecognised. When I attended an MS treatment centre for oxygen therapy, I was struck by the amount of banter and chatting that went on before and between treatments. Although the MS patients were physically more disabled than I was, they had stamina for socialising. But sessions always ran late and 45 minutes chatter before an hour and a half in the oxygen tank proved too much and, in the end, I gave up the treatments. By interacting with the well, or even with the differently disabled, there is always a risk of being caught in a situation from which there is no escape. Getting stuck with a self-absorbed talker, and feeling the energy ebbing away, leaves two options – being rude or suffering later. At the point of exhaustion, how many can turn heel and walk away from someone mid-sentence? Better to avoid such situations. Within the ME ghetto, 'Sorry, can't talk any more' is understood. The other person responds promptly by putting down the phone or walking away. There are no hard feelings for what in normal circumstances is peculiar, anti-social behaviour.

The severely ill and housebound

For those who are severely or chronically ill, or in the early, draining stages of this illness, seeking out and coping with a network of people, even supportive ones, may be too much.

Offering appropriate support to the severely disabled is a challenge doctors and politicians need to meet. There are so many people out there, bedbound, housebound and totally isolated, who are far too ill to attend meetings, to send and receive e-mails, or even to talk for more than a few minutes on the phone. Coping with more than one person at a time is beyond their limits. Marilyn, talking about her own son and others like him, says:

◆ It's a daily struggle. I admire David so much, I really do, and everyone with ME who's able to get up in the morning and just try to carry on. They have amazing courage. I think to even get up when you feel that ill, and you know, it's very hard to explain to someone how ill they feel, even to get up is a major achievement for them. So, yes, I have enormous respect for them and I just want them well now.

The challenge for all health professionals is to find ways of reaching out and helping extreme cases like these and of offering appropriate support to individuals who are stricken by illness.

PART 4

Coping with ME

CHAPTER **18**

Denial

> Denial functions as a buffer after unexpected shocking
> news, allows the patient to collect himself, and, with time,
> mobilise other, less radical defences.
> ELIZABETH KÜBLER-ROSS[1]

ME comes without an instruction manual. Not surprisingly, then, those who succumb to it run the gamut of coping strategies as they try to understand what has gone so badly wrong with their bodies. It takes a long time to come to terms with the complexity and comprehensiveness of the illness and to harness appropriate defences. Most people progress through the same sequence of stages:

- denial that there is anything seriously wrong;
- struggling on despite an obvious and relentless deterioration in health;
- hanging on to a normal existence;
- coming to terms, out of necessity, with chronic symptoms and a greatly restricted way of living.

For a sizeable minority who lie for years in darkened rooms, even these struggles to work out some sort of equilibrium are unavailable because they are too ill. They must build their lives again from a very low and different baseline. All the responses and coping strategies described here are understandable, even if some are counterproductive.

241

Strictly speaking, denial is not a coping strategy. It is a first reaction. Admitting to exhaustion, or to a delay in bouncing back from a bout of flu, rather than acknowledging the possibility of a serious, chronic illness, is a reasonable initial response. Besides, without a test to suggest a different diagnosis, it *is* the most obvious conclusion. But later, as the possibility of ME seeps in and symptoms match what is known of the condition, denial allows space and time to come to terms with a difficult and demanding illness.

Denial reflects the dread people feel about ME and, for those who already have it, the terror of a full-blown relapse. Of the 21 people interviewed, 17 either said that cancer would be an easier illness to deal with, or that they wished they had cancer instead of ME. They believed that with cancer they would be dealing with a different kind of illness with a name, a test, treatments, understanding, support from professionals, family and friends, and, most important of all, a prognosis.

One woman who had ME for seven years and was later diagnosed with ovarian cancer, subsequently undergoing a hysterectomy and radiotherapy, said:

- **Honestly, it was nothing compared with the ME. I wouldn't even rank the two together.**

Dawn, who had suffered a severe stroke which left her unable to walk or speak several years after she had ME, talked emotionally during one of the self-help classes about preferring another stroke than a ME relapse. With arm raised in mock volunteering, she said:

◆ 'Yes please. Me. Me. I'll take the stroke. I volunteer for the
stroke. I'd rather have another stroke and have to learn to
walk again and talk again than go through that again.'

Because of this fear, when ME-like symptoms strike, it is understandable to decide that it is something else. The chances
are that it *is* something else, the most likely alternative being
a self-limiting post-viral fatigue following an infection.

In my sample, only Bruce seemed to skip the stage of
denial, but he was pre-armed and well informed since he
had worked on cognitive behavioural programmes in the
past. In complete contrast, Chrissie, an artist who had had
ME for ten years, offers a story of persistent, blinkered denial
which finally tipped her into a much more severe form of the
illness. She was very ill in the early stages after a viral illness,
then gradually climbed back to a level of health at which she
could function – literally climbed because she would take
herself off to the mountains to walk, cycle, climb and paint.
Although she never regained her former level of fitness, she
built up her stamina over years until she could work, paint,
party and hike again. Never during this period of gradual
recovery and partial health did she seek a diagnosis nor
acknowledge the possibility of ME. Her illness was 'an inconvenience'. At the root of her behaviour, perhaps, were
comparisons with her super-fit boyfriend who sustained her
denial by dismissing and trivialising her pain and exhaustion, and by setting unrealistic physical fitness targets. And
so for years Chrissie pushed herself beyond her limits,
walking until exhausted, and socialising late into the night,
even after symptoms started to re-appear. It is surprising

that she lasted the course as long as she did, but she was extremely fit before she had ME and did not dip as deeply as some. But eventually she paid the price of denial. After ten years of behaving as if she was trivially unwell, she had a massive relapse. At the first self-help group meeting in California, pale and drained and obviously very ill, she could only just summon the energy to speak. Our group leader had asked us to introduce ourselves and to say what we hoped to get from the meetings. Chrissie wept as she said:

◆ This is me. I am it. I have CFIDS. It has taken ten years for me to say this. I am here because I am part of it.

Unlike Chrissie, most people with ME learn over time, and by trial and error, what they can and cannot accomplish without making themselves worse. Sweeping changes, modifications and fine tuning become a normal part of daily existence. As a result it is not always clear whether equilibrium and stability means real, long-term recovery or reflects an increasingly sophisticated skill in managing symptom levels. The surprising thing about Chrissie is that she tried none of this. She made no attempt to relate her behaviour to her symptoms – so each day was a fresh surprise or a new shock. Only by admitting that she had ME did she muster some control over the illness and set in motion the possibility of improvement. She kept a diary of symptoms and energy levels, and tried to live 'within the energy envelope'. After a couple of weeks she realised that there were patterns, such as predictable highs and lows in the day, and activities such as walking which exacerbated her symptoms. Instead of landscapes, she crayoned tiny beautiful postcards in child-like, sweetie colours. Most people with ME work out the necessity to do this sort of thing more quickly than Chrissie did, but others prefer to carry on without the constant monitoring and pacing which inevitably focuses attention on the illness.

I too went in for denial. When I first experienced relatively mild flu-like feelings, night sweats, and malaise following a viral infection in 1987, I decided to sweat it out at the gym. For six weeks I pumped iron, did aerobic classes and sat in the sauna in a stubborn effort to rid myself of the thing. I felt ill, and then more ill. Still I went to the gym, angry that the symptoms would not go away. Then one day I woke up feeling more ill than I can describe, and ill in a different way from anything else I had ever experienced. I could not get out of bed, nor did I for the next six months. I don't suppose I will ever know whether my manic sessions with the weights tipped a self-limiting post-viral fatigue illness into ME but with the wisdom of hindsight in those early weeks of illness, I would have stayed away from the gym.

Many others did as I did. They pushed their breaking bodies to the point where they broke. Most of the adults who took part in this project were extremely fit, physically active, health-conscious, and not completely poleaxed by severe onset and so they denied the possibility of serious illness for as long as they could – Alistair and Phil used to run marathons; Fraser trained intensively as a rugby player; Ray drove sports cars every weekend; Denise took part in swimming, yoga, aerobics and line dancing; Alison climbed mountains; Chrissie cycled. Their attitude was, 'I don't need to lie down under this.' And so, while May was sleeping for 12–14 hours a day and 'just existed' for a year, and while Janet was forced to take to her bed for six months, others, like Chloe, denied the possibility of ME for as long as they could keep going and sustain a semblance of normal life:

◆ I struggled on for about a year. I was working then, and eventually I was diagnosed with ME. I was off for six months and then I went back. I struggled on for years, to be honest, basically working and sleeping, no social life whatsoever. Then I went to part-time hours, about six hours a day, and still just sleeping and working. That was my life. I just pushed myself so much. My legs were heavy yet I'm the sort of person that I give my all, you know. I just kept pushing and pushing without realising it's the worst thing you can do with ME.

Ray's denial is typical of men with slow onset, who are not initially very ill, who never step inside a doctor's surgery, and do the macho thing of ignoring aches and pains. It did not cross his mind that he might be developing ME. Like Alistair and like Phil, his phenomenal energy made the possibility of chronic ill health something that he would never consider. This man was used to working hard and playing hard. He carried a huge workload as a sports car mechanic while simultaneously setting up his own business. At weekends he raced, driving the length and breadth of the UK to venues. Almost a year after the exhaustion set in, he finally went to his GP who reinforced Ray's idea of his own invincibility:

◆ 'There's nothing wrong with you. I can't get anybody in here that's fitter than you. Your name's in the local paper every couple of weeks winning this, winning that. You're doing so well. There's nothing wrong with you.'

Ray took time off work, then carried on again, 'just going downhill'. After another nine months a hospital consultant diagnosed chronic fatigue syndrome, but because the GP gave him no information about the condition other than advising him to take it easy, he carried on again. He continued to deny the possibility of chronic illness partly because he was left in the dark by his doctor and partly because he had too much to lose:

◆ I handed in my notice because everything was there. I had premises, and everything was in place. The banks were interested, and the enterprise people were like, 'This is the best business start we've ever seen. This is incredible. You just can't fail with this one.'

The other reason for denial was that his mindset about illness was completely wrong for dealing with ME:

◆ But I was always like that. I was always hell bent on, 'No, I'm just going to work through this.' Because that's the way I've done everything else in my life.

Ray lost everything. Just when he should have reaped the harvest of all his efforts, his health deteriorated so much that he had to stop altogether:

◆ My career's gone. If I went back to the motor trade I'd be starting all over again. Or I could start up again on my own but that would be mad because it's such a risk. I mean, even if I felt better, I could start up on my own and invest thousands and lose it because people relapse.

Now he says, 'I was silly really', but hearing his story, one can understand why he carried on.

Phil too was super-fit and training as a marathon runner before ME hit him. Like Ray, he had warning signs, but did the macho thing of ignoring them.

◆ I pushed myself harder and harder. The more fatigued I felt, the harder I would push.

Then one day he woke up ill – really ill. He rode the roller-coaster of work–rest–work for a long time still before admitting that things were seriously wrong. By this time he was so brain-fogged that when reduced to watching cartoons he 'couldn't work out whether it was the cat that was Tom or the mouse that was Tom', and so physically ill that he had to crawl on his hands and knees to answer the phone. Even then, one day, 'out of sheer desperation', Phil got up and went jogging. It was probably this final bloody-minded act of denial which pushed him into a severe and chronic form of the illness:

◆ I remember getting a few hundred yards and then collapsing and my heart felt like it was giving way. My breath was very very short. I thought, you know: 'I'm a marathon runner, how can this be?' I remember collapsing into a bath and lying in this bath for five hours in the freezing cold, unable to get out.

After trying to beat his illness into submission, Phil, aged 30, returned home to be cared for by his parents. He was bedridden, sleeping 18 hours out of 24, exhausted, emotional and suicidal.

Struggling on

Once upon a time there was something called convalescence, at least for the privileged few who could afford it. If you caught a chill or developed a fever, especially if you were 'delicate', you went to bed and were gradually nursed back to health. I remember, as a child, either I was well enough to go to school or I stayed in bed – not up watching TV or playing computer games, but under the covers with meals on trays and maybe a jigsaw puzzle as I recovered. If convalescence became fashionable again it would be just the thing for ME. Convalescence means it is acceptable to be ill, it means being looked after. It means resting until strength returns and a few steps, a first walk, can be managed without exhaustion. Nowadays this sounds like a passage from a Jane Austen novel – something far too wimpish. There are assumptions too about the effectiveness of this strategy, but anecdotal evidence suggests that those who get an early diagnosis and who rest thoroughly in the first months stand a better chance of an early and full recovery.[2]

Struggling on is different from denial. In denial, ill people pretend that they are not ill and press on, blinkered, refusing to look ME in the face, until a relapse or an intensification of symptoms stops them in their tracks. Often they hit rock bottom. When people struggle on, they do so in a bloody-minded way knowing, or strongly suspecting, that some-thing *is* seriously wrong. This is understandable because people *do* get up and go back to work with flu, or after surgery, and get away with it. But people with ME do not know that the harder they push, the more likely they are to propel themselves into a more profound version of the illness. Only with the wisdom of hindsight and armed with more information can they say, 'If only I had known, I would have rested more and I might not be so ill now.' Others struggle on because they are breadwinners and fight off the alternative of exchanging financial security for the sub-sistence living of disability benefits – assuming they are granted them. Others struggle on because they have young children or are single parents.

The single most important factor determining whether people struggle on or not is the severity of their illness. Those who kept going were, as a group, less severely affected by ME than those who did not. Several people said that, in retrospect, they were glad that initially they were so flattened that they had no option but to stop, rest and reassess their lives. Janet describes the severity of an illness so devastating that she had no option but to give in to it:

◆ I was overwhelmed. My immune system was overwhelmed probably because of all the pressures on me. I just got one virus, and then another and another and another, and that was it. Just right down as far as you can go. I just had to

succumb to this illness. I couldn't read for the best part of two years. I couldn't do anything really except listen to the radio and sleep. That's all I did.

Others are just about capable of keeping going, feeling appalling, forced to rest for half or two-thirds of every day in order to do what they want to do in the remaining hours, not out of ignorance or resistance but out of choice because they can not accept the losses and limitations. They are not ready to pay the price, because, in the context of ME, managing symptoms does not mean giving up an evening class, or sessions at the gym, or clubbing on a Saturday night, but accepting wholesale changes including perhaps the loss of a career, social life and all the other things which had absorbed their energies and interests up till then. Jamie *knew* he was ill and still he struggled on. He clung on to his teaching post, continued working for the local history group, gave talks, visited schools, and worked on his children's stories – all this despite the fact that his symptoms were severe.

◈ **I couldn't concentrate. I couldn't remember. I couldn't sleep.**

Jamie has not worked for 10 years. Yet one understands why he struggled on when he was already terribly ill.

This is how far people go to deny illness and hang on to their lives. Yet still some doctors might tell them that they don't try, that they lie down too easily under the illness. The truth is that they try too hard. They make themselves chronically ill by carrying on long after they should have stopped.

CHAPTER **19**

Hanging on in there

> Our culture is assembled around an idealised work ethic
> under which healthy, productive individuals are valued.
> FENNELL[1]

The distinction between struggling on and creating a deliberately curtailed life in which rest and activity are balanced
is a fine one. Making a conscious decision and taking steps
to hold on to part of a pre-ME existence involves acceptance,
coming to terms with a chronic illness, adopting deliberate
strategies, planned ways of living, adaptation and change. It
also requires a certain level of health and fitness to sustain
goals such as continuing at work, or continuing to function
as a homemaker. It is a testimony to the courage and determination of the people who tell their stories that so many of
them did manage to keep going, keeping a toehold in the
world of the well for as long as they could. Those who are
not bedbound play an intricate juggling game of doing as
much as they can to stay sane without knocking themselves
out or provoking a relapse.

Trying to maintain a plateau of semi-health while remaining in the world of the well is what Wells calls 'passing as
healthy'.[2] It is an understandable response in a world where
the expectations are that one remains healthy, energetic, and
productive, and where the old, the sick or the disabled may

be shunted into a siding without adequate resources or support. There are good reasons for trying to appear normal. Our society is uncomfortable with illness, especially chronic illness, as it prevents people from fulfilling the roles expected of them. Liam's distaste for defining himself as ill was such that he refused to go to bed during the day but slept in a chair, and even put on the television so that he did not drop off to sleep:

> LM: That suggests that you were unhappy with the idea of being a sick person?
> Liam: Who wouldn't be?

Keeping working

Unemployment makes people, the well and unwell alike, feel inadequate, useless and depressed.[3] Alistair understands the impact on his patients of having to give up their work:

> ◆ People are unable to work and probably get medical certificates saying debility, depression or something, and it's a tremendous blow to that person's ego that they can't work *and* they're off with something that no one believes in.

Which is why Fraser and others are determined to keep going, no matter what it costs in terms of increased symptoms and a longer recovery time. To give up work is too big a sacrifice.

Of the fourteen adults, twelve were in full-time employment when they became ill, one was in part-time work, and one the wife of a busy GP. Almost unanimously these people put work at the top of their priority list. They wanted to keep working, although, in the end, half were unable to do so. The exceptions were Chloe who missed her work as an audio-typist but regretted the loss of her social life even more, and Lizzie, who came to look back on ME as something positive which stopped her in her tracks when she was about to run over a cliff.

More men than women managed to keep working during the time they were ill and so 'passed for healthy'. Alistair, Fraser, Liam and Mike kept going throughout the period of their illness, whereas of the women only Fiona returned to do the same job by taking a short spell of sick leave and then working part-time until she was well enough for full-time employment. How can we explain these differences? Are there more pressures on men as breadwinners to keep working? Do men experience a greater loss of self-identity if they become unemployed or sick, and so fight harder to retain their jobs?

In my sample, the single significant difference in the equation of working or not working is the severity of illness combined with the level of support received during the early stages. Ray, Jamie and Phil also tried to keep working in the early stages of their illness, but failed because they became too ill. The men who managed to keep working reported an average disability level of 45 per cent at their lowest point, and are now either fully recovered or about 10 per cent disabled. Fiona was 60 per cent disabled at her worst and now 95 per cent recovered after a two-year illness. In contrast, Jamie was 80 per cent disabled at his worst point and is now

25 per cent disabled after ten years. Phil, the sickest of the men, was 95 per cent disabled for a long time and is now still only 50 per cent recovered after twelve years. Ray is functioning at 60 per cent of his former energy level, but seems to be deteriorating so his future is uncertain. Here, then is a more plausible explanation for the differences. The men, as a group, were less severely ill than the women, and were ill for a shorter time. Basically, those who could carry on working, did so. The rest gave up with regret, reluctance and at great personal loss.

The second, related factor is the level of support. Three of the four men who kept working had the support of a wife who took over all household and child-care responsibilities. Mike had the freedom of being unattached and said that he thought being single, being responsible for no one but himself, and being tolerant of a high degree of squalor was a factor in his own ability to keep working. The common factor here is that none of the men had responsibility for others. None had to run a household or care for children. They could invest their limited energy in getting through ME.

Liam epitomises the way men can keep working providing certain conditions are in place. Top of his list is the relatively moderate form of his illness compared with other people he knows about. But he describes other factors which helped him fulfil a determination to keep going:

◆ He was given a prompt diagnosis and so had no draining battles with either his GP or his consultant, both of whom accepted his illness as real and physical.

Shattered

- As head of department he had some control over his workload and a degree of flexibility in the way he worked so that he could re-organise his timetable, take a sabbatical, and postpone intellectually demanding work such as the writing of academic papers.
- He had the support of a loyal, competent wife who coped admirably with his illness.
- He was temperamentally suited to taking illness in his stride:

> I think because I'm not that reactive I could manage it better. I think if I'd been a more emotional person it would have been much more difficult to handle but I suppose in everyday terminology I'm fairly phlegmatic, sometimes annoyingly so I suspect. Although I can get angry, it's not very frequent in normal life and I certainly don't get emotional.

- He came from a background of Christian Science which, although no longer informing his own beliefs, still left 'a substantial residue.'
- He was committed to his department.
- He was committed to his work and loved its challenges. It was far more than a way of earning his living. Death from boredom was a less attractive option than soldiering on, even when ME symptoms caused discomfort, pain and exhaustion.

Alistair, Mike and Fraser describe exactly the same kind of conditions as Liam – the relative mildness of their illness in which pain and exhaustion rather than cognitive impairment were major symptoms; a fairly prompt diagnosis; lack of hostility from the medical profession; jobs which gave them some leeway and control; and the support of a caring wife.

Fraser's job as a firefighter may not sound the right kind of occupation for someone recovering from ME, but his days, he says, were very mixed with a lot of tea-drinking and sitting around the station as well as the mad scrambles when 'you were up to your neck in it'. His ability to keep going also owed a lot to the up-and-down nature of ME which meant that sometimes, but not always, the rush and scramble coincided with a high rather than a low in the diurnal rhythm of his days. Despite what it must have cost him to keep working, he reflects on his journey through the illness in a positive way:

* I can look back now and realise I was very lucky, you know. I was only really unwell for a couple of years.

Alistair gives the same sort of account of managing to remain at work. Here are the same common factors: a milder form of ME, a degree of control in the way he worked with colleagues who took over some of his workload for a while, no problems getting a quick diagnosis, and a wife who shouldered domestic responsibilities. He also shared with the other men a deep commitment to his job so that giving up work was an intolerable option compared with struggling on. But for Alistair, and for the other men, it was still very hard. Alistair behaved just like other patients in monitoring his progress and keeping a daily tally of his energy so he could judge how much he should do:

- I used to score each day out of 10. If I was 10 out of 10, I felt good, and then when I was really shitty and thinking about bed, I'd hover between maybe 2 or 3. I was aware that I was able to work – but only just.

I hope that I don't make it sound too easy for the four men who kept working. All describe their worst days as hellish, and for each of them, like Fraser, there were times when they thought they would have to give up:

- I wasn't going to lie down under it and start taking days off work. That was one thing I really decided not to do. And at my worst, about a year or two into it, there were days when I was really struggling at the station and there was almost one or two days that I really felt like booking sick and going home because I was feeling hellish. But then in the course of the day you would probably have a trough and then come back up again a wee bit. Rally during the day sometimes so it wasn't like a whole day feeling awful. It was very much a roller-coaster and you just hoped that if something happened it was in one of the peaks and not the troughs. There was a couple of times things happened and I really felt terrible.

Mike's life was reduced to the absolute basics so that he could work:

- I would go out, drive to work, and then literally just coming home, having something to eat and just lying on the couch watching TV, then going to bed.

He talks about his isolation, the loss of his social life, and how much he missed having a drink with his mates. Apart from work, there was just the one weekly visit to the pub:

> I made an effort to go out one night at the weekend and drink mineral water and that was it, and it didn't always work out because I wasn't always well enough to do that. I tried to make sure I was not staying at home seven days a week looking at four walls.

Looking back, he doesn't know how he managed to keep going. And for all the men the choice to keep working, as Fraser says, was a gamble which they may not have won:

> It wouldn't have been many per cent more and I wouldn't have been able to work. I must have just scraped through for a year and a half, maybe two years. For two years I was worried about being able to work, and it was a year after that that I felt comfortable at work.

So, did the four men pay a price by struggling on? Would they have got better faster and more completely if they had stopped? There are no answers to these questions. The facts are that the men made a good recovery, better than many of the others interviewed, despite the fact that they kept working – or possibly because they did so.

Unable to work

Most of the others tried to keep working, but even after they cut everything else out of their lives, they still could not handle the demands of long days, set hours, deadlines, and input over which they had little control. For those who could not carry on, cognitive impairment was a major feature of their illnesses.

Phil tried to hang on to his job as a youth worker after he became ill, but the job was arduous and stressful and involved commuting up and down the M8 between Edinburgh and Glasgow, often doing two consecutive eight-hour shifts in each place. During that time, he recalls having to pull off the motorway to gather the strength to continue his journey. He took time off, then tried various strategies to enable him to keep working – 'working part-time, working much shorter hours, getting a bit more support, stopping travelling through to Glasgow' – but to no avail:

> I knew there was something seriously wrong by this stage and I tendered my resignation on the grounds of ill health. It was me that just knew that I couldn't continue any more. I had a word with my employer telling him what I was intending to do. He was quite upset for me and saddened – but not half as much as I was.

Fiona tried to return to work as a university administrator after two bouts of flu from which she was not recovering:

> I went straight back to work. I was aware of just how tired I was. It was a real struggle to get through the work and

eventually I couldn't manage it. It was a feeling of being
overwhelmed.

The financial implications of not working

Most people are gutted when they are finally forced to turn
their backs on their work and careers. Suddenly a regular
salary is replaced by the form-filling and humiliation of the
benefits system; they have to adapt to subsistence living.
Without a career and a regular salary or wage, standards of
living plummet along with self-esteem. Phil says that some
weeks he has to choose between keeping warm and eating.

Ray, who previously earned a very good salary as a sports
car mechanic, is amazed by the amount of money he is
expected to live on now that he is sick:

◆ The dole is absolutely incredible. I got my first money a
   couple of weeks ago. That's been two and a half months to
   sort it out and they give me 50 pounds a week!

Before ME he had 'such a good lifestyle'. Now he cannot
make ends meet. Ray is just setting out on the benefits obsta-
cle course. Perhaps it is a good thing that he does not know
what lies ahead. People talk about their dread of applications
for Income Support or Disability Living Allowance (DLA) as
they face the surreal experience of filling in lengthy forms full
of irrelevant questions which were designed for people with
missing limbs, paralysis or mental illness. (My ill scientist
friend recently scrawled all over his form, 'There is not a
single question in this entire booklet which is relevant to the

way I feel with ME.') After the form-filling comes the scary, humiliating or irrelevant examination by a doctor who does not know you and may not know much about ME. The last one who assessed me wanted to talk about the virtues of Margaret Thatcher – I will never know whether I was turned down for DLA because of my medical condition or my political views. Finally there is the long wait for the apparently random results where the severity of symptoms and quality of life appear not to correlate with the outcome.

Alison was initially awarded DLA, then cut off, then forced to go to tribunal, given the mobility component but not the care component, then cut off again. This kind of drama is not unusual. She comments:

> The DLA is a big problem because they always assume you're lying, don't they? And they say, 'We disagree that you can't cook a main meal.' If you say that you can't, they say, 'Yes, you can.' I feel I've had to know how to go about getting it and how to jump through all the hoops they require you to jump through and I wouldn't have been able to do it if I hadn't been an articulate, confident, middle-class person with the help of this advice worker.

And if confident, articulate, professional people find the ordeal of applying for benefits too much to bear, what happens to the people who are not used to standing up for themselves or challenging the authorities?

In my sample, Alistair, Fraser, Mike and Liam all say that they would have lost the battle to keep working if their illness had been a couple of notches more severe. The others did try, but they were too ill and did not rest enough in the early stages, so their determination to carry on was finally thwarted when their symptoms overwhelmed and defeated them. In the stories told here, another myth is well and truly shattered. There is not a shred of evidence for a readiness to give up work, or relief to have an excuse to take time out from the real world.

Anderson reports that 27 per cent of participants forced themselves to keep working out of financial necessity and as a result paid the price in worsening symptoms. Despite being labelled 'shirkers', people with ME only give up work when they can no longer fulfil their workplace duties and when deteriorating health make physical and mental work impossible.

CHAPTER 20

OK, I'm ill: where's the pill?

Contemporary society has perpetrated a tremendous
number of myths about immunity, often grasping onto the
persuasive language of quick-fix healing in a desperate
attempt to thwart the failings of the body.
MUNSON[1]

An Action for ME survey of 500 members carried out in
1990 revealed that the average amount of money spent by
individuals searching for alternative cures in the UK is £900,
with one person spending over £16,000. Only 8 per cent felt
that they had wasted their money, while 53 per cent considered their expenditure a mixture of money well spent and
money wasted.[2] One response to these findings might be
that the placebo effect is a powerful one not to be lightly
dismissed. Also, after paying so much money for treatment,
there may be a reluctance to admit that there have been no
positive results. With regard to conventional drug treatments,
after compiling a formidable list of what was on offer,
Shepherd concludes that only a limited number of those
currently available seem to help some people with some
specific symptoms, while others are counterproductive or
have unwanted side-effects.[3] He describes an even longer list
of alternative and complementary approaches, concluding,
'Some seem to be of help, whereas others are nothing more
than pseudoscientific nonsense and a complete waste of
money. A small number (e.g., germanium) have turned out

to be positively dangerous, even fatal.'[4] The narratives here are in accord with Shepherd's findings. No one was significantly helped or dramatically made better by anything which they tried – either within the conventional or the complimentary repertoire.

People need to look for a cure – they need hope. It is because there is nothing that conventional medicine can offer that they keep on searching. If doctors do not understand ME, perhaps there is a complementary practitioner who will. Too ill to travel, nevertheless they take trains and planes to faraway places where treatment is promised. They spend their reduced incomes paying people who offer to make them better. The stories here tell of vitamins and supplements, diets, liquid oxygen, magnetic weights, crystals hung in windows and every conceivable new therapy hailed as a cure by the media, on the internet, in health shops, or on the ME grapevine. People are trying to crack the code without knowing which code they are trying to crack.

In this study, fewer men than women chased these rainbows. Either they were more rational, more macho or, as a group, not so seriously ill. Fraser read up on the disease, decided it was something more complex than he could deal with, and tried to carry on doing what mattered most – working. Mike tried evening primrose oil and royal jelly, but seeing no improvement gave up the search. Bruce stuck to fine-tuning his behaviour, and Alistair and Liam did nothing. Ray says:

◆ There's so many things people are trying, Chinese herbs and all the rest of it. I've done the herbalist. I've spent a couple of hundred quid. No step forward unfortunately.

Yet the two men who were most seriously ill, hunted just as hard as the women for a magic cure to make them better. Phil tells a story of a desperate and fruitless search for treatment:

◆ In the early years I still had some faith in the medical profession, or I wanted to have some faith in them so I stuck out with whatever I was offered and took it in the hope that they knew more about this than I did. Gradually it dawned on me they didn't.

And so he decamped:

◆ Into the weird and wacky world of alternative medicine … I tried colonic irrigation, iridology, acupuncture, sitting in pyramids, past life regression, homoeopathy several times, aromatherapy, nutrition, Chinese medicine, reflexology. That's just scratching the surface. Then tai chi, yoga – fair enough; 32 different treatments. My life savings of £10,000.

One of Phil's final 'acts of desperation' was, coincidentally, the same as mine – the ex-builder bloke from Glasgow who claimed to cure ME by deflecting electromagnetic and geopathetic stress by the strategic placing of bits of wood and metal:

◆ My logic hadn't completely gone out of the window. I was aware, at the time, that this looked like a rip-off, but while there was a one per cent chance, it was worthwhile.

As a reminder of his years of searching, and his gullibility, Phil keeps at hand the block of wood which cost him £70 and which, if placed near his taps, would 'block the harmful rays'. He sums up these desperate years as:

◆ There are some genuine, caring people who believe in their alternative therapies, and in some of the more accepted forms there may be something there for some people. There are also a lot of people who, while believing they are helping people, aren't and might actually be doing further damage. And there are sharks and charlatans in all different shapes and guises who prey on weak and vulnerable people.

Illogical acts are only a reflection of desperate situations. Even now, Phil has not stopped hoping and searching:

◆ Yeah. Out of absolute desperation, if somebody could convince me that 33 was the lucky number, I might still, even to this day, be tempted.

Like Phil, the women wanted to believe that somewhere out there was a solution. They were applying a problem-solving approach to a problem which could not be solved, like Fiona, who says, 'There must be *something* I can do.' Denise's story exactly mirrors Phil's – endless harmful prescriptions for antidepressants and painkillers prescribed by her GP before she retreated to complementary treatments. Like Phil, she spent a lot of money she could not afford on chiropractic, homoeopathy, acupuncture, reflexology, massage and, finally, psychoanalysis. One can only understand and sympathise.

It is very hard to come to terms with the fact that currently there *is* no proven, effective treatment for ME. Denise was previously active and fit, a 'sporty person . . . a busy person who lived life to the full'. Surely, then, she could conquer this illness in the way she had previously tackled her life – head-on:

◆ I had lots of friends. I'm the bright and bubbly one who got them all organised. 'Right, where will we go, what will we do?' I would stir them.

It took her a long time to realise that she could not organise her way out of ME.

Among the young people I interviewed, five out of seven have first names which begin with J. Among the men, four out of seven have names which begin with 'N'. Does this make first name initials a factor in the development of ME? OK, it's laughable, but so are many other of the suggestions, treatments and cures which people fall for.

Fruitful searches

Three women did not search in vain. They did not find a magic pill, nor a quick end to the ME symptoms, but they would probably say that they found something more valuable and long-lasting.

May, who had helped her husband with his newsagents business and then his milk round for most of her working life, read up on natural remedies as her 'zombie state' receded. Like Lizzie and Janet, she talks of ME almost as a necessity – as something which had to come along and stop her in her tracks and make her look again, and look hard, at the way she was living. Her studies confirmed what she intuitively felt about the illness, and gave her a different perspective and a new insight into what happened to her:

◆ Very often it [ME] can be triggered off with a virus that you don't ever get over properly. But that's not the whole story. I think that it is the trigger rather than the cause, and I don't think pumping alien drugs into one's bloodstream does any good. I think you need to look for natural remedies. I mean, at one stage I actually sort of thought that it's, not exactly, nature's way of returning the body to what it should be. That's what I believe about my case now. I was fighting nature too much by pushing my body too far, physically and mentally probably, and it's a bit like if someone has a bad lifestyle and they have a heart attack – it's a warning. I feel it's a warning from nature. You're not doing yourself any good. Re-evaluate your life.

Her interest in alternative treatments eventually led to her homing in on the subject of world mythologies.

◆ I would say I've found an open-minded spirituality. I started understanding the spirit of nature. I think that helped me. I started to get myself in tune with natural cycles because everything in nature has a cycle and I think that has helped me. I've taken more than a passing interest in world mythologies. It's interesting to see how people use the mythical cycles and different beliefs to find their own way of understanding nature.

Now she is studying part-time for a degree in anthropology.

Janet was ill for 17 years from the age of 52. As she read about and experimented with alternative therapies, she became immersed in Buddhism and Eastern philosophies, experimented with diets, became an expert in dowsing and, like May, made radical changes to the way she lived and the way she thought about health and illness. The transcript of her talking about those years is a description of a slow metamorphosis:

⬧ I believe in reincarnation and karma, I believe things are meant. I believe in synchronicity and accept everything which has happened to me. I find my life enriched immeasurably because of what I believe. Those years were not lost to me because they altered my thinking. I'm a much stronger person now. My life is enriched and enhanced by what I have gone through.

Janet is still ill, but she describes her life as positive, exciting and fulfilling. Lizzie was combining professional dance training with a degree in English when she became ill:

⬧ I was training to be a dancer of a very high standard plus choreography and essay writing. Dancing all day and studying. The drop-out rate was huge.

She lasted for four months before collapsing with what she describes as 'a life crisis in which you get physically knocked.' Over the next two years, she went from therapy to therapy, finding in each something positive, regarding the process as a personal learning curve. She did art therapy, encountered the art of massage in a Steiner therapeutic centre, consulted nutritionists, added supplements to her diet, practised transcendental meditation and yoga, and worked for two years with a healer. What she learnt was to let go:

◆ Ah, I'm ill. I stopped fighting. I'd been fighting the whole time. This fight, this arrogance that I had a concept of what my life was going to be about and nobody was going to change it.

From dance she moved finally to massage which she describes as:

◆ A form of movement therapy ... Half way through every massage I would be in heaven, like dancing with this other person, and in tune with them. I knew somewhere that this was how I was going to get well. This massage is going to help me get well because it's bringing me back down to reality. I knew it was the right thing for me to do.

I love Lizzie's story of recovery and self-discovery. It proves that searching for a cure can lead off in new and unexpected directions. The headless chicken run after pills and therapies can change into a positive, thoughtful and life-enhancing journey. Lizzie describes herself as stuck with a mind-set which would have made any significant improvement in her health and well-being almost impossible. The door to recovery opened only when she let go and created a different way of living:

◆ I had an illness called ME. I think I had a real crisis. You get given a situation and you work with it as best you can. Now I feel like I'm very blessed.

These stories must be set in the context of all the others. Lizzie and May were among those least seriously affected by ME and so perhaps were able to harness levels of energy not available to others. Perhaps the relative shortness of their illnesses was a contributing factor. Perhaps the natural course of the illness was in their favour like a tide that had already turned. Janet, in contrast, was extremely ill and although she is better, it is relative to a very low base-line and she seems to have reached a plateau. What she describes is not recovery but a slow process of adaptation, learning, acceptance and change which has lasted almost two decades. It would be condescending to suggest that anyone can get themselves on an upward, healing spiral if they listen to their bodies and be more conscious about their way of living. Two women found a way of recovering and moving forward, and one found peace and spiritual fulfilment. This leaves eighteen men, women and young people who either worked out a different way of dealing with ME while it lasted, or who are still ill. And many of those who are ill are still searching.

CHAPTER 21

Still life: a different way of living

> Life in itself was worth living. And always unpredictable. It
> was a question of living what there was of it on a different
> basis of expectation. One could, she had learned, get used
> to things.
> COOPER[1]

> When you are sick, surrender does not mean giving up
> hope of renewed health. Rather, it means accepting all the
> circumstances of your life, including present sickness, in
> order to move beyond them.'
> KANE[2]

Acceptance

Acceptance is not the same as giving up. It is a positive adaptation to chronic illness. After all, trying to carry on as before is like pushing a boulder up a slippery mountain with one finger – it won't go. In the long term, acceptance is probably the only way to nudge forward the possibility of recovery.

It is a long haul from the onset of puzzling symptoms which might be ME to the endgame which is a resigned, angry or sad acceptance that this is how things are going to be. The signposts and stages along the arduous and emotional journey to acceptance are clearly documented in the narratives told here. First, for as long as they can convince themselves, people fight hard to deny the possibility that they might have something as frightening and disabling as ME. Then, once they admit the possibility, they begin the search for something or someone to make them better. When that fails, they take increasing responsibility for their illness, making changes in the way they live so that they can manage, cope and live within its limits. After that, it's a question of balancing gains and losses in order to make slow progress or to maintain an equilibrium. A minority recover sufficiently to turn their backs on the whole dreadful experience, except when occasional symptoms return. The rest have to get on with it. Some are quick and efficient in working out a new, limited life agenda. Some are inwardly resourceful and quietly determined. Others fight harder and for longer, taking years to accept the necessity for finding a balance of rest and activity that will put them on an even keel. In the end, there is no choice but to arrive finally at 'an uneasy peace with our disease'.[3]

The king of acceptance in the narratives here is Bruce who applied his knowledge of cognitive-behavioural programmes to timetabling a strict and disciplined structure for his own recovery. On the surface his story seems a simple case of a man accepting his illness, working out a way not only of coming to terms with it but also of overcoming it by adapting his life completely to its demands. The method worked for him. He was able to draw a graph of his recovery projectile. But it wouldn't necessarily work for others because Bruce was not severely ill at onset and temperamentally he was suited (as much as one can be) to the regime he imposed on himself. He relates an anecdote about a man who came to one of his classes. After sitting through the first session, listening to advice about energy envelopes, goals, diaries and targets, he said: 'Frankly, I'd rather get a life.' And while acceptance is an efficient coping strategy, it can also be a wafer-thin layer over days of despair. Bruce's almost instant acceptance of illness, his insight into knowing not to fight it, and his minutely orchestrated approach to recovery has paid off. But at a price of tough self-discipline and loneliness. And I know from our intimate conversations how difficult it has sometimes been for him.

If Bruce is the king, then Ruth is without doubt the queen. Amongst ourselves, we women in the self-help group in California called her the 'queen of suffering' because of the skills with which she managed and accepted an almost intolerable level of pain. Ruth, suffering from severe fibromyalgia, lived in a spiritual community where, as well as her own two modest rooms, there was a communal dining room and a place for worship and meditation. She was rarely well enough to get to either. Unlike Bruce, she did not need a timetable or an agenda because after two decades of pain she was used to listening to her body and knew instinctively how much she could do. Ruth needed 12 pillows to manage a meditation session. She could not walk. She could not watch TV because it was too much of a sensory overload. Even some pieces of music and certain books and radio programmes were impossible because she did not have the strength to cope with powerful emotions. Ruth had considered taking her life. Instead, she has accepted it. With her wisdom and deep spirituality, she has found the inner strength to reinvent suffering as a necessary and positive experience.

Part of acceptance is not talking about ME. The illness is not going to go away in a few weeks, nor is there going to be any significant change in the short term so there is little point in issuing constant health bulletins. It's hard not to tell everyone how you feel every couple of hours, especially when you are going through a rough patch, but it gets boring and tedious for everyone else. Dr Darrel Ho-Yen suggests giving people a once-a-day score, say 4 or 7 out of 10, and then nothing more.[4] It is a common perception that the chronically ill are preoccupied with their illnesses but the overwhelming majority of people said they adopted a deliberate strategy of not talking about their health, either with close family and friends, or with outsiders. Bruce said that when he met new people, he never told them that he was ill. Knowing any attempt at explanation would be energy-draining and counterproductive, he only made himself available during good phases of the day, and for periods of time which he was confident he could manage. This way he avoided the barriers that went up whenever he mentioned ME, and dealt with his illness in the way he wished – in private.

But what about the young people? How do they accept the losses of a life hardly begun? The answer they give, like the adults, is that they have to. Not one of them was self-pitying, nor asked why this had happened to them. As Josh said:

◆ I haven't exactly got any choice in the matter but to get on
with it. Why waste energy being angry?

This is what, in essence, each of them said. They could not afford to spill energy on anger or regret. For Chris, putting a lid on emotion is part of adaptation and acceptance:

◆ All my energy is spent holding myself together and
sometimes I feel like crying and breaking down, but then
I think if I do I am not going to be able to pick myself
up again.

Marilyn suggests that one reason why her son David was
able to cope with ten years of profound disability, including
four years when he could do virtually nothing for himself, is
that he knows no different:

◆ I get the impression that he doesn't appear to have any
resentment about being ill. I think it's because he's been ill
for so long and I genuinely believe that he's forgotten what
it's like to be well. I know it's sad but I don't feel there's any
resentment, I really don't.

For five out of the seven young people the beginning of
illness is almost impossible to pinpoint because they experienced so few years of 'normal' childhood before they became
unwell so that any yardstick of 'healthy' or 'normal' has all
but disappeared. Acceptance is based on hazy notions of an
ordinary life.

The young people's anger and bitterness is reserved for
the professionals who treat them so carelessly and harshly.
While they yearned for open and informed dialogues about
their illness with doctors and teachers, they did not want to
dwell on ME by talking about it all the time. Kirsty says of
the young people's support group:

◆ People don't want the stigma attached to a group where we talk about our symptoms. We talk about, sort of, the normal side of the small segment of our lives.

Talking about her 20-year-old son, Marilyn said several times, 'Very rarely, very very rarely' do they talk about ME. But she also said:

◆ When he does want to talk to me, I will just drop everything and I will listen because I know when he does want to talk to me, he really does want to talk.

When David finally decided, after many years, to join a young persons' support group, he did not tell his mother. This was one small act of independence which he managed for himself.

Driving back from my interviews with the young people I cried as I put myself in their shoes. There they were, aged 14, 16 and 20, housebound, stuck with mum and dad and the cat, missing out on an irreplaceable period of growing up, their education halted, their social life dead – and still they were brave, stoic, even funny. Their emotional pain sometimes pushed through the surface, and most wept as they talked. They accept because they have no choice but to accept, but still their courage is amazing.

Facing the future: four years on

You don't get over this kind of experience when you start to feel better. You grow beyond it.
JOSH

We are becalmed by the lack of an ending. The stories in these pages document how truly awful it feels to live with an uncertain future. ME, an illness which is both acute and chronic, leaves us in a constant state of waiting. We are passengers on a journey waiting for the train to come. Some of us doubt that there is a train. The questions we ask go round and round in loops until we accept their futility. Will we improve? Will tomorrow be better than today? Will there ever come a time when we are ourselves again?

The waiting is different for those who remain severely ill, for those who have reached a plateau where good and bad spells come and go with apparent capriciousness, and for those who are fully or partially recovered. Where recovery remains totally elusive, even after many years, there is only an hour-by-hour managing and clock-watching getting through each day. Progress, if it comes, is glacial. Others – probably the majority – can predict to some extent what they can do and how much energy they dare release without exacerbating their symptoms, but even then the trip wires can appear suddenly and arbitrarily in front of them. They live cautious lives, ekeing out reserves, playing a perpetual game of suck-it-and-see, trying not to run on empty. Of course, sometimes one decides to do it and be damned; live today and pay for it tomorrow. Even for the self-styled lucky ones who have regained most or all of their previous health, ME leaves a residue in terms of curbs and restrictions. Whereas once they would have strode boldly forth, now, perhaps for a second, they hesitate. And for every one who has had ME, the most desperate legacy is fear. The fear of a major relapse casts its shadow – faint for some and menacing for others – over each and every life.

It is now four years since I started this project. I wanted to know what had happened to the subjects. Had any of them made a significant recovery? Many had stayed in touch with me since the original interviews; others I contacted by e-mail and letter.

From the replies came some good news – even some very good news. What most people said was that they were very slowly improving although no one had found a magic bullet of a cure nor had suddenly and miraculously got better. But they were better than when I talked to them four years ago and for many the quality of their lives had improved. Here are some of their replies. I hope that they offer hope and consolation to every one of you ill with ME who is reading this book, wondering if your life will ever change. It can and it does.

THE WOMEN

Chloe

I have a beautiful little boy – and as you know I just never thought this would be possible. He's fifteen months old now! It's a dream come true. He makes everything worthwhile, especially when I'm having a bad day. My mum and dad have been helping out a lot so I've been really lucky. But I must admit sometimes I wish I could do more with him. Our new house is lovely. We have a fairly big garden so even on a bad day, if I can't get out, it's lovely just to sit outside for a bit and get some fresh air. J loves running about in the garden. It's great watching him learn new things all the time. I had been keeping fairly well but then I had a very busy two months with four big birthdays to celebrate, including J's first, then J's christening and moving house in the same weekend, so I am back to taking things really easy.

Janet

My life has moved on well since your visit. We have been offered a site and caravan to buy in Ardnamurchan with permission to build a kit-framed house. Having the prospect of living in such a beautiful place has given me a tremendous boost.

Since your visit, I have gradually improved. I put this down to vitamin and mineral supplements. I have also found great benefit from yoga and swimming and a small amount of hill walking. Perhaps the biggest help has been a spiritual one. I received, and then trained to give healing as a Reiki Master and find great benefit from both.

Away from the village with its busy main street and busy supermarkets, and my commitment to young grandchildren, I am revelling in minimal traffic, narrow roads and no street lighting. I enjoy creating a garden when the weather is conducive and I have enough energy.

This is a completely suitable lifestyle for me and I feel myself, at the age of 70, to be in control of my ME at last.

May

When we met, I was pretty much on an even keel and able to take preventative steps at the first sign of a flare-up. This has fortunately continued. Compared with others, I consider myself very lucky.

Life is far more positive for me now. My husband is happier and fitter than he has been for years because he has given up the doorstep milk deliveries. He has become a human being again instead of the robot he was turning into. Apart from the obvious benefits for him, this has been a great help to me because – prepare to be amazed – I am now an undergraduate at Edinburgh University doing an MA part-time. This is the end of my third year and if I pass the exams, I will have six of the eleven modules required for Honours, and my director of studies is talking about postgraduate possibilities. I guess it's not bad for a 53-year-old who left school with one 'O' level. I'm really enjoying it and find a self-fulfilment I would not have had if I'd gone to university when I was younger. I am grabbing the opportunity with both hands.

Alison (and Peter)

In the last four years we have both had a very gradual improvement in our ability to do things. The improvement has been slight but significant. We both started to play the piano again to the extent that we were able to participate in an Edinburgh Festival summer school last year, albeit in a very limited way. We haven't been able to do it again this year. We still draw up our groceries on a rope and get them delivered when we can. We don't have to lie in a darkened room so often, and our periods of pain and extreme fatigue are not so frequent.

In the last year I have been determined to have adventures, realising at last that I might have ME for the rest of my life. They have included a walk on the coast (about half a mile), a trip to the family clan in Ireland, two trips to London where a friend let me stay in bed 20 hours a day and to sally forth and see life for the other four in the company of my trusty three-legged aluminium stool.

Peter made a day trip to Glasgow to listen to a piano master class; practised half an hour a day for six weeks in preparation for a 45-minute piano lesson then collapsed for a week; since then he realises he can't practise consistently enough to make any progress. However, he has started to compose a short piece of music and one day hopes to finish it.

Lizzie

Four years on and I certainly feel that I have more energy and more focus in my life. I was working full-time at the time of the initial interview, but still had to have quite a lot of space, and time for the odd nap. Now my days are very full and I am constantly challenged to 'fine-tune' my ability to relax and not store up too much tension. But now I can feel restored after a ten-minute break rather than the two hours that it used to take. It is too easy to cut off and live according to what my head is telling me I can do rather than the reality of what is possible, and to think 'I'm fine' when in fact I am upset about something. So I try to tune in to how I am feeling, both physically and emotionally. Over time this has had a positive accumulative effect – a bit like a muscle that gets stronger with use.

The other thing that has helped me greatly is to have a partner who perhaps sees me more clearly than I see myself, and can tell when I am in danger of overstretching myself. This has been a blessing as it is hard to try to stay sane and keep your feet on the ground all on your own. My work too is very helpful as I have to be grounded and present to be effective, and the environment is peaceful which allows for a meditational quality to be there as I work.

As a footnote, I have realised in the past two years just how important a role candida played in my debilitation of energy. I think it preceded my breakdown by a number of years and has still not completely cleared up. But in recognising its significance I have started to focus in on it more, and it is gradually improving.

Chrissie
In the summer of 1999, I had a very serious relapse relating to a relationship I was in where I received a lot of criticism. I was conducting my life as if I had an inconvenience rather

than a chronic illness. After three years, I have recovered about 40 per cent of my pre-relapse functionality.

Treatments that helped me when I could barely sit up include intravenous vitamins, called Myers Mix, twice weekly for a year, and Doxepin, an antidepressant, for sleep. I was cared for by a lay Buddhist monk whose modern conveniences included a radio and a bicycle. I learned to allow only positive people in my life and watched only happy movies.

After six months, I started telephone counselling sessions, and did a little walking and yoga stretches. I took a lot of hot baths and created a 48-hour rotation diet to relieve pain. When I was able, I watched clouds, tended a little 'plant hospital', and sketched.

One year ago, I started taking several 'potions' that have made a big improvement in my health. Micohydrin is a powerful antioxidant containing silica hydride. I also take colloidal minerals, Knox Gelatine for joint inflammation, and one half teaspoon of baking powder to help create an alkaline body environment that viruses don't like. On alternate days, I drink either carrot juice or a green juice consisting of spirulina, romaine lettuce, Swiss chard, red cabbage and parsley. I take digestive aids and acidophilus daily, and give myself B12 shots once or twice a week.

I tend to have more energy when I avoid prescription drugs – I am phasing out a tranquilliser called Klonopin for sleep. Other things that hinder energy are caffeine, chocolate, sugar and, of course, stress. Meditation practice and re-ordering my life to reduce stress help greatly. Also, examining my life daily to eliminate co-dependent behaviours reduces stress. I work on loving myself exactly as I am – a life's work in itself.

Today, I am venturing into a new relationship with a professional artist. We paint together two days a week (I can work for about three hours at a time), and we make music with musician friends. I am assuming more household chores (I have a helper come two to three times per week) and make the highest priorities of keeping emotionally well-balanced and pacing my activities.

Marilyn
In truth, I have found it very difficult to get my head round this. I suppose it is all too painful; I am sure you will know what I mean.

The last four years have seen a steady improvement in David's health, with the usual ups and downs, of course. However, he is still only at the stage where he can work between one and two hours per day. Now into twelve years of ME, my feeling is that without the intervention of some new treatment, this is as good as it is going to get for him. At the age of 25 he does have youth on his side to be able to benefit from any new treatments that hopefully will come along within the next few years. In the meantime, it is a case of 'care and maintenance'. My view, gained from much experience of ME, is that the best I can do for David is to provide a home environment which is as stress-free as possible; ensure there is good healthy food in the house – organic where possible; and give him care and support when it is needed. Mostly David is very positive and rarely complains, and I have the utmost admiration for him in the way he copes with this relentless illness.

I, as a single parent, am mostly coping too. In the first few years of ME I surrounded myself with people, support groups and information, all in a desperate attempt to make sense of the complexities of this illness. There comes a time though when it is vitally important, as a long-term carer/supporter, that one develops interests outside the home and the illness, and to have someone in your life who you can chat to about all things *but* ME. A long-term carer gives so much emotionally, it is important you have someone in your life who can give you just a bit back in return. For this I am indebted to my friend 'A'.

As for the future, it is a parent's duty to provide their children with roots and wings. I have provided David with roots; I hope successful research will provide him with the wings he needs to fly the nest and start living a normal life. In the meantime, it will be my pleasure to support and care for him until that magical moment arrives.

THE MEN
Phil
Since meeting you some four years ago, I believe that my health has improved significantly, as a result of consulting with Dr David Smith in Essex, who believes that ME is a neurological condition, which is treatable with the administration of a variety of antidepressant medications at low dosage, combined with a lifestyle programme. It is always tricky to objectively measure my percentage of improved health, but I would estimate that if I had 50 per cent health when you first interviewed me that this has increased to 75 per cent health today. The symptomatic improvements include:

- More lucidity, improved cognitive functioning;
- Improved memory;
- Improved mood;
- More energy;
- Reduced muscular pain.

I do not believe that I have, as yet, been cured of my ill health but I am certain that Dr Smith's ongoing regimen has been of tangible benefit to me.

Most of what I am doing cannot be classified as paid work – although I hope that this situation will change in the months and years that lie ahead! Nevertheless, I do a little paid work as a sort of personal care assistant for someone severely affected by ME and make pocket money from car boot fairs at weekends!

Alistair

For the last year I have had no symptoms even with stress and viral illnesses. As I said to you, my attacks were often preceded by halitosis, and two weeks ago, just prior to a holiday, my wife said I had bad breath. I immediately became introspective and searched for symptoms – but none came! I am fully active, enjoying golf, climbing and skiing, and regard myself as 'cured' – but I still keep 'looking over my shoulder' as I never quite believe it is away.

Liam

Eventually it is possible to forget, for long stretches of time, that ME disrupted my life for several years, but now and again events bring back that period and evoke painful memories.

Now, I am left with the occasional physical reminders of extreme tiredness and debilitating weakness, and a reaction to the noise of fans or to long train journeys, but mostly I feel much as I did before the illness. At last, I can dig the garden, even shovel gravel, without having frequent, long rests. Thinking back, I realise that ME affected not only me, but my family. ME has destroyed some families, others may emerge stronger, but the feelings associated with the illness cause great strains, which change the course of family life. ME makes you depressed, selfish, exhausted, intolerant, angry for no apparent reason, and generally difficult to live with – often for many years. I am left with profound gratitude that my own family patiently supported me through the experience and that, as the symptoms abated, we were able to build a more normal life again.

Mike
I have to say I am improved in health. I have reached the stage where I can take gentle cardiovascular exercises three or four times per week, usually 20–25 minute sessions, and I try to swim about four times per week, managing sessions of up to 30 minutes. However, these are more of an excuse to go for a sauna or visit the steam room. The exercise has built up from about August last year when I started doing a few lengths of the 20-metre pool. I built up to it gradually but I have put on a bit of weight which contributed to the decision to try exercising, after discussing it with my GP (a fellow sufferer). I did not take any supplements: it was more of a gradual build up of health, particularly as my immune system recovered. I felt that if I could exercise it would help me further in building on the recovery.

I still have to be careful with my health. I can occasionally take alcohol without any major problems, but if I take even 1–2 units every day over a period of two weeks then I start to notice a deterioration in my health with the pain in my legs returning. I also notice that if I do catch any virus going around (it doesn't always happen now my immune system seems to be as strong, or nearly as strong as before the ME), I have a return of my ME symptoms on top of the illness and my recovery time is not always as quick as with 'healthy' people, but it is only a few extra days at most.

I suspect I will never be 'clear' of the disease but I have been successful at managing it by being conscious of things like stress levels. I can control almost all stress except workplace stress but if I let that build up then, in common with a lot of people, I get ill when a 'bug' is going around.

THE YOUNG PEOPLE
Kirsty

'It had no beginning and certainly has no definable end.' I wrote that eleven years ago. ME is unfortunately no fairytale with a Happy Ending (at least, until a cure is discovered). I live in hope, otherwise I would have given up a long time ago.

I am, however, nearer to that fairytale in a slightly different sense. My knight in shining armour came along – and he hasn't run away yet, from me or my ME! It takes incredibly special people to truly understand ME and I have been blessed that he does, along with my mother and father who without a doubt have been there for me throughout.

Acceptance is one of the key things to making a recovery – accepting you have ME (that took me a while), doctors (that took them even longer!), other people accepting you have it. And without a cure, acceptance and support are the best substitutes. I am now learning to manage my ME – learning to live within my limitations and to make the most of each day. It's a bit like Michael J Fox and his fight with Parkinson's disease: 'If you were to rush in this room right now and announce that you had struck a deal – with God, Allah, Buddha, Christ, Krishna, Bill Gates, whoever – in which the ten years since my diagnosis could be magically taken away, traded in for ten more years as the person I was before, I would, without a moment's hesitation, tell you to take a hike.'

ME has enriched me and all those who suffer are survivors of this illness, not victims. ME and 'my knight' have taken me quite literally to places I had never thought possible!

Chris

For a long time my state of health was very poor and deteriorating. After seeing a private ME specialist who followed the Tietelbaum Protocol my health improved. Low adrenal hormones and thyroid levels were corrected but my temperature still remains low and I get chilled very easily. My chronic insomnia and pain were addressed. My energy levels and pain improved with better sleep. But I still cannot get the full solid 7–9 hours that are said to be needed for recovery. I take multiple medications but with some I either react to them or gain a tolerance to them over a short period of time so they no longer work.

For years I battled with chronic diarrhoea and with pimples occurring in my mouth while I was eating. After a fight for funding, the Health Board agreed to fund allergy treatment in Great Ormond Street in London. The treatment is called Enzyme Potentiated Desensitisation (EPD), a vaccine that contains antigens to foods, inhalant and chemicals. I am halfway through the three-year treatment protocol and my body seems less sensitive to things now. I have read that EPD has a beneficial immune modulating effect on the body, which helps in the recovery of ME. I am also following a specific carbohydrate diet for the treatment of chronic diarrhoea.

As my health has improved, I have been able to do a couple of evening classes and volunteer at a local charity shop once a week. I was lucky enough to be given a garden allotment and I get a lot of pleasure from this. I get help with the digging. I still have to pace myself and can get crippling back pain from doing a little weeding and there are of course ME pains that come out of the blue without a cause. The worst thing about this illness for me is the loneliness that comes from being in the house most of the time and the lack of energy and money for socialising.

I would say I am just over 70 per cent well, but this is a fragile 70 per cent which can be upset really easily.

Jessie

I have come a long way in the last few years. I have been studying for a BSc (Hons) in Chemistry and am about to go into my final year. I decided to take a year out last year and managed to work part time in quite a physical job. This did me the world of good because it let me improve my physical fitness with a lot less stress, and my condition definitely improved.

There's no magic formula, but I've found that gentle exercise like swimming and walking helps, along with trying to minimise and manage stress. The support of my family and friends has been invaluable. I am still aware of my limits but try to gradually extend them. Sunshine helps a lot – just a shame I live in Scotland!

Hopefully, I'll finish my degree next year, and then take it easy for a while. I plan to work part-time and save up to go travelling. I'm not 100 per cent yet, but I'm definitely getting there. It seems to take forever, but I try to stay positive, I know I'll get there eventually.

Josh

Four years ago, the GP told my parents to prepare themselves for the possibility that I might not live. I was bedbound. I had no life.

After three years of very slow improvement, and ups and downs, it is only in the last year that there have been significant changes in the quality of my life. I live independently in my own flat. In a limited way, I am mobile. I have passed my driving test. In August I started college studying for one 'A' level and have an understanding tutor who lets me attend a full-time course in my own flexible time, and this way, so far, I keep going.

I am happier now although I am not like my peers in terms of freedom, choices, health and energy. I enjoy life in my bubble. Things are a million times better than four years ago but it is a case of being content with what I have. That doesn't mean I do not long for what I could have. I feel that I have lost the life that I might have had, but for now I am satisfied and hope that things improve further.

My way through is not to think about ME. When I do, I get upset and angry; what's the point in banging your head against a wall? I concentrate on my work when I am fit enough. I see friends when I can. I grit my teeth and get by, not dwelling on what I have lost. You don't get over this kind of experience when you start to feel better. You grow beyond it.

THE AUTHOR
Lynn Michell

Today (because 'finally' is tempting fate) I am free from the burden of monitoring and worrying about my every move. My health is stable *and* I have become canny and selfish enough to manage my days so that I won't upset the ME apple cart. The processes of acceptance, adaptation and getting better are inextricable; don't ask me which comes first because it's impossible to say.

There was a watershed called ME. Before it, I lived life at full throttle, not 'driven', but blessed with bags of energy. Last year I held on to one last thread of that life when I agreed to teach psychology to MSc students. But the 9am start, the fluorescent lights, the bleak seminar room, the three hour stint defeated me. This year I said, 'No.' My refusal means a final letting go of work which brings status, self-identity – and an income.

Now I run workshops for women, teaching creative and therapeutic writing. The setting is a calm, meditative room in an alternative centre. The time is mid-day. Natural light pours in the large windows. The wise, wounded women surprise and delight me with their writing, sharing, support and bonding. A two-hour session doesn't tire me, rather it enriches, renews and satisfies. Once a week I go to the art college to cut stained glass. I am a beginner, cack-handed among the proper art students, but what fun to mess about and with no other aim than to create something beautiful.

When I'm tired I go to bed; often I fall asleep. I try not to rush or set deadlines. I am slow in the mornings and fairly useless in the evenings. My mother used to call me Speedy Gonzales. All that has gone and in its place, when I am focused, there is a quieter, slower, more reflective way of living. I am not saying that being fast caused ME, but being slow is the only way for me to control it. I need solitude and space and silence – for most of the hours of every day. As much as I can, I have filtered out people and behaviours that make me tense, tired and unwell to avoid the payback later. This is my normality. Sometimes it feels lonely, often it feels good, but mostly it feels necessary.

Where once my life was disrupted by illness almost to non-living, now it flows again.

ME/CFS: The research perspective

Myalgic Encephalomyelitis/Chronic Fatigue Syndrome (ME/CFS) is a serious, often disabling, chronic illness. Researchers in the United States have reported that quality of life of patients can be seriously disrupted, and the social consequences – as regards employment, relationships, financial security, future plans, personal worth – can be severe. Similar findings have been reported by Australian researchers who, in fact, found that people with ME/CFS had more dysfunction than those with multiple sclerosis. Yet, despite the seriousness of the condition for large numbers of people, comparatively little serious biomedical research has been undertaken. The situation has been complicated by the fact that – like most 'syndrome complexes' – the wide disease category contains a variety of sub-groups, with specific causes and symptoms requiring particular treatments. For some people, illness will have been triggered by an infectious process, but in others the onset might have been insidious or activated by an environmental event. Given the extent of the problem – the recent report by the Chief Medical Officer of England estimates that ME/CFS affects between 0.2 and

0.4 per cent of the United Kingdom population, with similar levels in USA and Australia – it is now clear that biomedical research should be a major priority.

Despite the general lack of interest in funding biomedical research into this illness, there are nevertheless some promising lines of enquiry. There is now a growing body of data showing that specific immunological factors may underlie the condition: for example, in some people with ME/CFS, an increased frequency of autoantibodies to certain insoluble cellular antigens has been shown. In Brussels, Professor Kenny De Meirleir is certain that ME/CFS is a disorder of the immune system. He has produced a substantial body of work showing a dysregulation of the 2-5A synthetase/RNase L antiviral defence pathway and has developed a constellation of markers that might be useful for the characterisation of sub-groups of patients. The damage caused by these small molecular fragments is not visible on standard blood tests because they interfere with receptor signalling and specific cell surface ion channels and proteins that can only be assessed by specific and sensitive assays. A good example of this in ME/CFS patients might be thyroid function where, despite normal thyroid hormone blood tests, ME/CFS patients may be hypothyroid because of the way in which Rnase L fragments interfere with thyroid receptor behaviour.

There is also evidence that cardiovascular abnormalities may have a role in perpetuating the illness in some people with ME/CFS. A research group at the Chronic Fatigue Syndrome Cooperative Research Center in New Jersey has reported lower cardiac stroke volumes in CFS patients compared to controls, suggesting that low cardiac output may have a role in the post-exertional fatigue characteristic of myalgic encephalomyelitis and that such abnormalities cannot be explained by de-conditioning alone. Also, recent work in the UK on physiological responses to incremental exercise in ME/CFS has found a hypo-dynamic cardiac response to heart rate exercise. In support of this, recent work from Israel on the ability of the cardiovascular system in CFS patients to withstand stressors confirms a view that the abnormalities to cardiovascular system plays a significant role in the exacerbation of symptoms in ME/CFS. One of the most common complaints in ME/CFS is a range of cognitive symptoms and some researchers have looked at the possibility that these are associated with a mild encephalopathy. One study using magnetic resonance imaging (MRI) of the brain found abnormalities in a subset of ME/CFS patients and, indeed, most abnormalities on these scans were found to occur in ME/CFS patients with no major psychiatric disorder. At present, there is ongoing work investigating the relationship between brain ventricular volumes and ME/CFS, and these studies and others using functional MRI and positron emission tomography (PET) are likely to provide answers to some of the central nervous system problems that ME/CFS sufferers have to face every day of their lives.

Research has also confirmed abnormalities of the choline pathway in the brain of people with this illness, with evidence of high levels of free choline in the occipital cortex. Our own ME/CFS research work in the Peripheral Vascular Diseases Research Unit at the University of Dundee which is funded by MERGE has indicated further abnormalities to a specific choline pathway in small blood vessels of ME/CFS patients, exhibited as a significant sensitivity to acetylcholine delivered across the skin. These results contrast with comparable research on people with other medical conditions, such as cardiovascular diseases, diabetes and hyperlipidaemia, where an impaired response to acetylcholine is the norm: the phenomena in ME/CFS may well be related to inhibition of endothelial expression of the enzyme, acetylcholinesterase. There are, however, some paradoxical findings for we have also confirmed the work of others showing high levels of oxidative stress in these ME/CFS patients, a biology consistent with insensitivity to acetylcholine. These findings were seen only in people with ME/CFS and not in either organophosphate-exposed patients and Gulf War syndrome patients, despite the fact that they have an illness that is often indistinguishable from ME/CFS. There is, I believe, sufficient evidence to speculate that ME/CFS might well be a type of vascular disorder, not in the strict sense that includes atherosclerosis or vasculitis, but as a special manifestation of impairment to the layer of cells lining the blood vessel wall, namely the vascular endothelium. Evidence for this hypothesis comes from numerous reports of vascular dysfunction in ME/CFS visualised in the central nervous system by SPECT and PET imaging, with one study highlighting specific blood flow abnormalities at the level of the brain stem. These reports, along with the various studies of orthostatic intolerance – an insidious drop in blood pressure on being upright – have never been explained and our new work on dysfunction of the vascular endothelium goes some way to addressing this vacuum.

In further MERGE sponsored research, Dr Kennedy at the University of Dundee has recently discovered abnormalities to neutrophils in ME/CFS patients when compared to age and sex-matched controls. This particular finding is potentially very important: the role of neutrophils is to phagocytose and destroy infectious agents, including virally infected cells and tumour cells, and the phenomenon may be related to persisting infection. Since Professor De Meirleir's findings in relation to dysregulation of the 2-5A synthetase/RNase L antiviral defence pathway may be linked to disturbances to many pathways including oxidative stress, lipid peroxidation and specific disorders of cell function, it is reasonable to conclude that there is a great deal of harmony between the current research efforts along a variety of fronts.

While all the findings reported above could well be the result of a persistent immune challenge, much more work needs to be done to confirm and extend the findings of biomedical research worldwide so that a sound working model of the pathogenesis of ME/CFS can be developed. At the present time, the diagnosis of ME/CFS is based on clinical case definitions and there is no indubitable diagnostic marker for the condition. Nevertheless, there is mounting evidence across a range of biomedical specialties that physiological abnormalities can be found in sub-groups of ME/CFS patients. What are needed now are the resources – and, importantly, the will – to resolve the biomedical basis of the condition: as the report of the working party on ME/CFS to the Chief Medical Officer of England in January 2002 stated,

'Research is urgently needed to elucidate the aetiology and pathogenesis' of this illness – for the benefit of patients and their carers everywhere.

DR VANCE A SPENCE

CHAIRMAN

MERGE (MYALGIC ENCEPHALOMYELITIS RESEARCH GROUP

FOR EDUCATION AND SUPPORT)

The Gateway

North Methven St

Perth

PH1 5PP

Scotland

UK

www.meresearch.org.uk

References

Introduction

1 Wells SM, *A Delicate Balance: Living Successfully with Chronic Illness*, Insight Books, Plenum Press, New York and London, 1998, p1

2 Bergner M, Bobbitt RA, Carter WB, et al, 'The Sickness Impact Profile: Development and final version of a health status measure', *Medical Care*, 19, 1981, pp787–805

3 Sontag S, *Illness as Metaphor*, Penguin, London, 1983, p67

4 *ibid*, p58

5 Munson P (ed), *Stricken: Voices from the Hidden Epidemic of Chronic Fatigue Syndrome*, The Haworth Press, London and New York, 2000, p3

6 *ibid*, p4

7 Boseley S, 'I tried to pretend I didn't feel as ill as I did', *Guardian*, Society, 12 January 2002

Chapter 1 – What is ME?

1 A Report of the CFS/ME Working Group: Report to the Chief Medical Officer of an Independent Working Group, February 2002

2 Anderson JS and Ferrans CE, 'The quality of life of persons with Chronic Fatigue Syndrome', *Journal of Nervous and Mental Disease*, 1997, 185, 6, pp359–67

3 Burne J, 'A Battle for the Weary', *Times Online*, 2 October 2002

4 Shepherd C, 'Conference Diary' in *Perspectives*, 80, Summer 2001, pp6–11

5 Fukada K, et al, 'The chronic fatigue syndrome. A comprehensive approach to its definition and study', *Annals of Internal Medicine*, 1995, 123, pp74–6

6 Jason LA, Richman JA, Rademaker AW, Jordan KM, Plioplys AV, Taylor RR, McCready W, Huang C-F and Plioplys S, 'A community-based study of chronic fatigue syndrome', *Archives of International Medicine*, October 1999, 159, 18, pp2129–37

7 Wells SM, *A Delicate Balance: Living Successfully with Chronic Illness*, p1

8 Kenney KK, 'Wichita study reveals much about who has CFIDS', *The CFIDS Chronicle*, November–December 1998, p25

9 Carpman V, 'San Francisco prevalence study alters CFS profile', *The CFIDS Chronicle*, Winter 1997, p82

10 Jason LA, et al, 'A community-based study of chronic fatigue syndrome', pp2129–37

11 Shepherd C, *Living with ME*, Vermilion, London, 1994, p39

12 Vojdani A and Lapp CW, 'Interferon induced proteins are elevated in blood samples of patients with chemically or virally induced chronic fatigue syndrome', *Immunopharmacol Immunotoxicol*, 1999, 21, 2, pp175–202

13 Behan PO and Haniffah BAG, 'Chronic fatigue syndrome: a possible delayed hazard of pesticide exposure', *Clinical Infectious Diseases*, 1994, 18, 1, S54

14 Burke J, 'Children suffer stress over their "love-lives"', Education Unlimited, *The Observer*, 29 October 2000, p7

15 Shepherd C, *Living with ME*, p30

16 Smith A, 'The scale of perceived occupational stress' *Occupational Medicine*, 2000, 50, 5, pp294–8

Chapter 2 – Telling it how it is

1 Anderson JS and Ferrans CE, 'The quality of life of persons with Chronic Fatigue Syndrome', pp367

2 Berne K, 'Running On Empty: The Complete Guide to Chronic Fatigue Syndrome', Hunter House, Alameda, CA, 2000

3 Clauw DJ, 'The pathogenesis of chronic pain and fatigue syndromes, with special reference to fibromyalgia', *Medical Hypotheses*, 1995, 44, pp369–78

4 Hans Selye, *The Stress of Life*, McGraw Hill, New York, 1956

5 Bell DS, Robinson MZ, Pollard J, Robinson T, Floyd B, *A Parent's guide to CFIDS*, Haworth Press, New York, 1999, p78

6 Hinds GME, et al, 'A retrospective study of chronic fatigue syndrome', *Proceedings of the Royal College of Physicians of Edinburgh*, 1993, 23, pp10–14

7 Ray C, et al, 'Coping and other predictors of outcome in chronic fatigue syndrome: a one-year follow-up', *Journal of Psychosomatic Research*, 1997, 43, p405–15

8 Bombardier CH and Buchwald D, 'Outcome and prognosis of patients with chronic fatigue and chronic fatigue syndrome', *Archives of Internal Medicine*, 1995, 155, pp2105–10

9 Wilson A, et al, 'Longitudinal study of outcome of chronic fatigue syndrome', *British Medical Journal*, 1994, 308, pp756–9

10 Shepherd C, *Living with ME*, p121

Chapter 3 – How bad can it get?

1 Bell DS, *ME: The Disease of a Thousand Names*, Pollard Publications, Lyndonville, New York, 1991, p185

2 Report of the UK Government Chief Medical Officer's Working Group on CFS/ME. Children and Young People, *The Key Points*, a specialist publication edited and produced by Tymes Trust, Ingatestone, Essex, 2002

3 Colby J, 'Chronic Fatigue/ME', *Special Children*, February 2002, p1

4 Dowsett EG and Colby J, 'Long-term sickness absence due to ME/CFS in UK schools: an epidemiological study with medical and educational implications', *Journal of Chronic Fatigue Syndrome*, 1997, 3, p2

Chapter 4 – Reaching parts other illnesses don't reach

1   Kane J, 'Be Sick Well: A Healthy Approach to Chronic Illness', Oakland CA, New Harbinger, 1991, p3

2   Wells SM, *A Delicate Balance: Living Successfully with Chronic Illness*, p135

3   Shepherd C, *Living with ME*, pp154–5

4   Wetherell A, 'Cognitive and psychomotor performance tests and experiment design in multiple chemical sensitivity', *Environmental Health Perspectives*, 1997, 105, 2, pp495–503

5   Michiels V, de Gucht V, Cluydts R and Fischer B, 'Attention and information processing efficiency in patients with chronic fatigue syndrome', *Belgian Journal of Clinical and Experimental Neuropsychology*, 1999, 21, 5, pp709–29

6   Michiels V and Cluydts R, 'Neuropsychological functioning in chronic fatigue syndrome: a review' *Acta Psychiatrica Scandinavica*, 2001, 103, 2, pp84–93

7   DeLuca J, 'Neurocognitive Impairment in CFS', *The CFS Research Review*, 2000, 1, p3

8   Slotkoff AT and Clauw DJ, 'Fibromyalgia: When Thinking Is Impaired', *Journal of Musculoskeletal Medicine*, 13, 9, Sept 1996, pp32–6

9   Munsen P, Stricken: *Voices from the Hidden Epidemic of Chronic Fatigue Syndrome*, pp1–2

10 Hyde BM, 'The Definitions of ME/CFS: A Review', in Hyde MD, Goldstein J and Levine P (eds), *The Clinical and Scientific Basis of Myalgic Encephalomyelitis/Chronic Fatigue Syndrome*, The Nightingale Research Foundation, Ottawa, 1992

11   Shepherd C, *Living with ME*, p121

Chapter 5 – An illness without a diagnosis

1   Sontag S, *Illness as Metaphor*, p61

Chapter 6 – Not real or acceptable

1   Sontag S, *Illness as Metaphor*, p61
2   Patarca-Montero R, Antoni M, Fletcher MA and Klimas NG, 'Cytokine and other immunologic markers in chronic fatigue syndrome and their relation to neuropsychological factors', *Applied Neuropsychology*, 2001, 8 (1), pp51–64
3   Chaudhuri A and Behan PO, 'Fatigue and the basal ganglia', *Journal of the Neurological Sciences*, 2000, 179, pp34–42
4   McCully KK and Natelson BH, 'Impaired oxygen delivery to muscle in chronic fatigue syndrome', *Clinical Sciences*, 1999, 97 (5), pp603–8
5   Lane R, 'Chronic fatigue syndrome: is it physical?', *Journal of Neurology, Neurosurgery and Psychiatry*, 2000, 69, p280
6   Paul L, Wood L, Behan WM and Maclaren WM, 'Demonstration of delayed recovery from fatiguing exercise in chronic fatigue syndrome', *European Journal of Neurology*, 1999, 6 (1), pp63–9
7   Bou-Holaigah I, et al, 'The relationship between neurally-mediated hypotension and the Chronic Fatigue Syndrome', *Journal of the American Medical Association*, 1995, 274, pp961–7

8   Scott LV and Dinan TG, 'The neuroendocrinology of chronic fatigue syndrome: focus on the hypothalamic-pituitary-adrenal axis', *Functional Neurology*, 1999, 14 (1), pp3–11

9   Spence VA, et al, 'Enhanced sensitivity of the peripheral cholinergic vascular response in patients with chronic fatigue syndrome', *American Journal of Medicine*, 108, pp736–9

10 Michiels V and Cluydts R, 'Neuropsychological functioning in chronic fatigue syndrome: a review', pp84–93

11 Wolfe F, American College of Rheumatology Annual Scientific Meeting, November 1998, San Diego, California, reported in *The Fibromyalgia Times*, Winter 1999, 4, 1

12 Ferguson E, 'The power of positive thinking', People, *Observer*, 26 November 2000, p16

13 Showalter E, *Hystories: Hysterical Epidemics and Modern Culture*, Columbia University, New York, 1997

Chapter 7 – The psychiatric fallacy

1   Sontag S, *Illness as Metaphor*, p39

2   Williams M, 'Considerations of some issues relating to the published views of psychiatrists of the "Wessely School"', *ME Research UK*, 2000, pp 61–3

3   Sontag S, *Illness as Metaphor*, p61

4   Russell J, *The Fibromyalgia Times*, Winter 1999, p5

5   Feinmann J, 'It's good to talk', Society, *Guardian*, 28 June, 2000, p2

6   Laing RD, *The Divided Self*, Penguin, London, 1966

7   Wells SM, *A Delicate Balance: Living Successfully with Chronic Illness*, p134

8   MERGE Report, 'Unhelpful Council', Report on the CMO Working Group Report, 2002

9   Jason LA, et al, 'The politics, science and the emergence of a new disease: the case of Chronic Fatigue Syndrome', *American Psychiatrist*, 1997, 52, 9, pp973–83

10 Royal College of Physicians, Psychiatrists and General Practitioners. Report of a joint Working Group of the Royal College of Physicians, Psychiatrists and General Practitioners: Chronic Fatigue Syndrome, Cathedral Print Services, London, 1996

11 MERGE Report, 'Unhelpful Council'

12 Shepherd C, *Living with ME*, p41

13 Williams M, 'Considerations of some issues relating to the published views of psychiatrists of the "Wessely School"', p5

14 *ibid*, p6

15 *ibid*, p36

16 Bradley L, *The Fibromyalgia Times*, Winter 1999, 4, p1

17 Sontag S, *Illness as Metaphor*, p59

Chapter 9 – Consulting rooms

1   Daly E, Komaroff AL, Bloomingdale K, Wilson S and Albert MS, 'Neuropsychological function in patients with chronic fatigue syndrome, multiple sclerosis, and depression', *Applied Neuropsychology*, 2001, 8, 1, pp12–22

2   Dowsett B, 'Spot the difference: ME, depression and unhappiness', *Tymes Magazine*, 32, Summer 2000, pp15–17

3 Reported in Wells SM, *A Delicate Balance: Living Successfully with Chronic Illness*, p30

Chapter 10 – Young people and doctors

1 Speight N, 'Child protection on the Chief Medical Officer's working group agenda', *The Journal of the ME Association*, 72, Autumn 1999, p8
2 Fish L, 'Panorama: Mistreatment of children with ME', *Interaction*, 32, January 2000, p5

Chapter 11 – Alternative practitioners

1 Spiegel D, *Living Beyond Limits: New Hope and Help for Facing Life-Threatening Illness*, Random House, London, 1993
2 Diamond J, 'Quacks on racks', Comment, *Observer*, 3 December 2000
3 Munson P (ed), *Stricken: Voices from the Hidden Epidemic of Chronic Fatigue Syndrome*, p13
4 Shepherd C, *Living with ME*, p294
5 Stoler DA, 'Alternative medicine: miracle cure or malpractice?', *The Providence Phoenix*, 25 June 1999, p10
6 Wells SM, *A Delicate Balance: Living Successfully with Chronic Illness*, p155

Chapter 14 – Family and friends

1 Michell L, 'Loud, sad or bad: young people's perceptions of peer groups and smoking', *Health Educational Research: Theory and Practice*, 1997, 12, pp1–14

2   Michell L and Amos A, 'Girls, pecking order and smoking', *Social Science and Medicine*, 1997, 44, 12, pp1861–9

Chapter 16 – ME in the family: parents and siblings

1   Sloper P, 'Needs and responses of parents following the diagnosis of childhood cancer', *Childcare Health and Development*, 1996, 22, 3, pp187–92

Chapter 17 – Seeking support

1   Schweitzer A, *Out of My Life and Thought*, Holt, Rinehart & Winston, New York, 1949, p194
2   Campbell B, *The CFIDS/Fibromyalgia Toolkit: A Practical Self-Help Guide*, Bruce Campbell, Personal communication, July 2002, (www.cfidsselfhelp.org/books; www.cfidsselfhelp.org/artcl)
3   Glajchen M and Magen R, 'Evaluating Process, Outcome, and Satisfaction in Community-based Cancer Support Groups', *Social Work with Groups*, 1995, 18, 1, p2740
4   Witter D, 'When you are among friends', *Arthritis Today*, 1996, 10, 5, pp41–6

Chapter 18 – Denial

1   Kübler-Ross E, *On Death and Dying*, Macmillan, New York, 1969
2   Shepherd C, *Living with ME*, p118

Chapter 19 – Hanging on in there

1 Fennell PA, 'The four progressive stages of the CFS experience: A coping tool for patients', *Journal of Chronic Fatigue Syndrome*, vol 1, no 3/4, pp69–79
2 Wells SM, *A Delicate Balance: Living Successfully with Chronic Illness*, pp138–9
3 Achieson D, *Independent Inquiry into Inequalities in Health*, The Stationery Office, London, 1998

Chapter 20 – OK, I'm ill: where's the pill?

1 Munson P, *Stricken: Voices from the Hidden Epidemic of Chronic Fatigue Syndrome*, p14
2 Shepherd C, *Living with ME*, pp294–5
3 *ibid*, p201
4 *ibid*, p293

Chapter 21 – Still life: a different way of living

1 Cooper L, *Fenny*, Virago, London, 1965
2 Kane J, *Be Sick Well: A Healthy Approach to Chronic Illness*, New Harbinger, Oakland, CA, 1991, p155
3 Weil A, *Spontaneous Healing: How to Discover and Enhance Your Body's Natural Ability to Maintain and Heal Itself*, Fawcett Columbine, New York, 1995, p251
4 Ho-Yen Do, *Better Recovery from Viral Illnesses*, Dodona Books, Inverness, 1994

Further reading

Self-Help Books

Living with ME
Dr Charles Shepherd, *Vermilion, 1999*
Dr Shepherd is Medical Advisor to the ME Association. This
book is available from the ME Association.

Better Recovery from Viral Illnesses
Dr Darrel Ho-Yen, *Dodona Books, 1999*

Chronic Fatigue Syndrome: A Treatment Guide
Erica Verrillo and Lauren Gellman, *Quality Medical Home Health
Library, 1998*

*Chronic Fatigue Syndrome – a victim's guide to understanding,
treating and coping with this debilitating illness*
Gregg Charles Fisher with Stephen E Straus, Janet Dale, Paul R
Cheney and James M Oleske, *Warner Books, New York, 1987*

*Chronic Fatigue Syndrome (CFS) (PVFS) (ME): Your Questions
Answered*
Mrs Frankie Campling and Dr John Campling, *The Erskine Press,
revised edition, 2001*

A Delicate Balance: Living Successfully with Chronic Illness
SM Wells, *Insight Books, Plenum Press, New York and London, 1998*

Finding Strength in Weakness: Help and Hope for Families Battling CFS
Lynn Vanderzalm, *Zondervan Publishing House, 1995*

The Hidden Viruses within You
Dr Bruce Duncan, *Viroprint, Wellington, New Zealand, 1994*

Knowing ME: Women Speak about Myalgic Encephalomyelitis and Chronic Fatigue Syndrome
Caeia March (ed), *The Women's Press, London, 1998*

A Life Worth Living – A practical guide to living with myalgic encephalomyelitis
Dr Michael Midgely, *Overton Studios Press, Colwyn Bay, 1995*

Lives Worth Living – Women's experience of chronic illness
Veronica Marris, *Pandora, London, 1996*
This books deals with the experiences of women with a range of conditions, including cancer, ME, lupus, multiple sclerosis, diabetes, epilepsy and heart disease.

ME – Chronic Fatigue Syndrome: A Practical Guide
Dr Anne Macintyre, *Thorsons, 1998*
Available from the ME Association.

ME – The New Plague
Jane Colby, *First and Best in Education Limited, Peterborough, 1996*

The ME Tips Collection
Zoe Williams, *1999*
Available from the ME Association.

Running on Empty
Dr Katrina Berne, *Bloomsbury Publishing, 1992*
Foreword by Dr Anne Macintyre

Stricken: Voices from the Hidden Epidemic of Chronic Fatigue Syndrome
Peggy Munson (ed), *The Haworth Press, London and New York, 2000*

Zoe's Win
Jane Colby, *Dome Vision, 2001*

Medical Books and Reports

Betrayal by the Brain - The neurologic basis of chronic fatigue syndrome, fibromyalgia syndrome, and related neural network disorders
Jay A Goldstein MD, *The Haworth Medical Press, New York, 1996*
This is a very heavy read and I would advise any patient to approach it with caution.

The Canary and Chronic Fatigue
Majid Ali, *Life Span Press, 1994*

Chronic Fatigue Syndrome/ME – House of Commons Research Paper, 1 December 1998
Available online at the House of Commons library,
www.parliament.uk/commons/lib/research/rp98/rp98-107.pdf

Chronic Fatigue and its Syndromes
S Wessely, M Hotopf and M Sharpe, *Oxford University Press, 1998*

Chronic Fatigue Syndrome
Jesse A Stoff and Charles R Pellegrino, *HarperPerennial, Tacoma WA, USA, 1992*

Chronic Fatigue Syndrome
SE Straud (ed), *Marcel Dekker, New York, 1994*

Chronic Fatigue Syndromes: The Limbic Hypothesis
Jay A Goldstein MD, *The Haworth Medical Press, New York, 1993*

The Clinical and Scientific Basis of ME/CFS
Byron Hyde (ed), *The Nightingale Research Foundation*

Clinical Management of Chronic Fatigue Syndrome (Clinical Conference, American Association of Chronic Fatigue Syndrome)
N Klimas and R Patarca (ed), *The Haworth Medical Press, New York, 1995*

A Companion Volume to Dr Jay A Goldstein's Betrayal by the Brain – A Guide for Patients and their Physicians
Katie Courmel, *The Haworth Medical Press, New York, 1996*

ME: The Disease of a Thousand Names
Dr David S Bell, *Pollard Publications, Lyndonville, New York, 1991*
For an updated version of this book, please see *The Doctor's Guide to Chronic Fatigue Syndrome* below.

The Doctor's Guide to Chronic Fatigue Syndrome: Understanding, treating and living with CFIDS
Dr David S Bell, *Addison Wesley, 1993*
This is an updated version of *The Disease of a Thousand Names.*

Enteroviral and Toxin Mediated Myalgic Encephalomyelitis/Chronic Fatigue Syndrome and Other Organ Pathologies
John Richardson, MB BS, *The Haworth Medical Press, New York,* 2001

ME/CFS/PVFS: An exploration of the key clinical issues prepared for health professionals
Dr Charles Shepherd and Dr Abhijit Chaudhuri
Available online at www.meassociation.org.uk.

NHS Services for People with Chronic Fatigue Syndrome/ME
National Task Force
Available from www.westcareuk.org.uk.

A Report of the CFS/ME Working Group - Report to the Chief Medical Officer of an Independent Working Group. January 2002
Available online at www.doh.gov.uk/cmo/cfsmereport/index.htm.

Outline for Development of Services for CFS/ME in Scotland – Report of the Scottish Short Life Working Group
Available online at
www.scotland.gov.uk/pages/news/2003/02/SEHD307.aspx.

Report from the National Task Force on CFS, PVFS and ME, 1994
National Task Force
Available from www.westcare.org.uk.

Report on Survey of Members of Local ME Groups, December 2000
Dr Lesley Cooper

Understanding ME
Dr David G Smith, *Robinson Health, 1989*

Personal Stories

Diana's Story
Deric Longden, *Corgi Books, 1993*

Jailbreak - A slow journey through Eastern Europe
Gill Suttle, *Scimitar Press, 2001*

ME and My Ducks
Linda J. Howard, *Janus Publishing, 1996*

One Step at a Time
Julie Sheldon, *Hodder and Stoughton, 2000*
Ten-year-old Georgie Sheldon, aspiring ballet dancer, was
suddenly diagnosed with a malignant brain tumour from which
she recovered – only to be affected by ME.

A Year Lost and Found
Michael Mayne, *Darton Longman and Todd, 1987*

Other Books Which Some People May Find of Interest

Climbing Out of The Pit of Life
Dr Darrel Ho-Yen, *Dodona Books, 1995*

Directory for Disabled People (8th Edition)
Ann Darnbrough and Derek Kinrade (eds), *Prentice Hall, 1998*
Outlines the range of statutory services available and covers
subjects such as aids and equipment, independent living, carers
and caring, mobility, education and legislation. Around 400
organisations and self-help groups are listed, and other sources of

information are provided. Useful information is also available from:

National Information Forum
Post Point 10/11
BT Burne House
Bell Street
London
NW1 5BZ

Tel: 020 7402 6681
Fax: 020 7402 1259
Website: www.nif.org.uk/

Illness as Metaphor
Susan Sontag, *Penguin, 1983*

Relaxation

Website: /www.relaxation.clara.net/
Provides independent reviews and information on guided
relaxation tapes – a non-profit site to help people find good tapes
on the web (similar idea to book review pages of magazines).
No tapes are sold but attempts are made to identify the cheapest
supplier for each tape.

Unwind (Relaxation)
Dr Darrel Ho-Yen *Dodona Books*

Resources

ME or CFS Organisations: UK

Action for ME and Westcare – www.afme.org.uk/
National ME/CFS patient support organisation that
works jointly with The ME Association on various issues.
Together with The ME Association, the National ME
Centre and Westcare UK, they are founder members of
the ME/CFS Alliance. A registered charity since July
1989, Westcare UK provides consultations in Bristol and
Gloucestershire with professional advisers/counsellors for
people with PVFS/ME/CFS. Offers residential rehabilitation courses. Holds a specialist medical reference library.

Association of Young People with ME – www.ayme.org.uk/
Free information, advice and support to people with ME,
aged 25 or under, their families and friends.

ME Association (UK) – www.meassociation.org.uk/

MEACH Trust – www.meach.org

MEActionUK – www.godot.connectfree.co.uk/

MERGE (ME Research Group for Education and Support) –
www.meresearch.org.uk

National ME Centre – www.nmec.org.uk

This is a registered charity established to provide both inpatient and outpatient care for patients with chronic fatigue syndromes of all types. Offers counselling and is also linked to the Regional Neurological Unit at Oldchurch Hospital where facilities exist for inpatient assessment and rehabilitation. Contact: National ME Support Centre, Disablement Services Centre, Harold Wood Hospital, Romford, Essex RM3 9AR; Tel: 01708 378050

Overton Trust – www.ostrust.freeserve.co.uk/

The 25 per cent ME Group –

www.btinternet.com/~severeme.group/

The 25 per cent Group deals specifically with people severely affected by ME.

Tymes Trust – www.youngactiononline.com/

The trust supports young people with ME and their carers. A registered charity, it works in partnership with www.youngactiononline.com; Contact: Tymes Trust, PO Box 4347, Stock, Ingatestone, Essex CM4 9TE; Tel: 01245 401080; Fax: 01245 401080

Young Action Online – www.youngactiononline.com/

Website for children with ME/CFS, parents and education run by Jane Colby. Young Action Online has joined forces with the Tymes Trust (*see above*) and you can register with the Tymes Trust at the website.

ME or CFS Regional Support and Information Sites in UK

BRAME – ds.dial.pipex.com/comcare/brame/

CHROME – ds.dial.pipex.com/comcare/chrome/

CHROME (Case History Research On Myalgic Encephalomyelitis) is a registered charity set up in 1994 with the aim of identifying as many severely disabled ME sufferers as possible in the UK and monitoring the course of their illness over a period of 10 years. From this study a body of statistical data will be collected and analysed which will supplement medical research in important ways. Contact: CHROME, 3 Britannia Road, London SW6 2HZ; Tel: 020 77363511; Fax: 020 77363511

Clywd ME Support –
  www.dialspace.dial.pipex.com/town/parade/ni30/ME/
Mid-Wales ME Group – welcome.to/midwalesmegroup
Scot ME – www.scot-me.fire-bug.co.uk/
Sheffield ME Group – www.sheffieldmegroup.co.uk/
Shropshire & Wrekin ME Support: Shropshire & Wrekin
  ME Support Group – www.shropshiremesupport.org.uk/
Support ME Hampshire – uk.geocities.com/smepetersfield/

Europe

CFS Information International – www.cfs.inform.dk/
Czech Republic CFS Association –
  www.htconnect.cz/advitam/
European CFS/ME and FM Organizations –
  home-13.tiscali.nl/~mesti/infopaginas/organisaties.html
Fatigatio e.V. – Das Chronic Fatigue Syndrome CFS (German
  ME/CFS Association) – www.fatigatio.de/
French CFS Association – asso.nordnet.fr/cfs-spid/
Italian CFS Association – www.salutemed.it/cfs/
ME Fonds (in Dutch) – www.mefonds.nl/

ME Platform (in Dutch) – www.me-platform.vuurwerk.nl/
Swiss CFS Association – www.verein-cfs.ch/

USA

About.com – CFS/ME – www.chronicfatigue.about.com/
Beat CFS and FMS – www.beatcfsandfms.org/
CFIDS and FMS Support Group of Dallas and Fort Worth,
    Texas – www.virtualhometown.com/dfwcfids/
Co-Cure – www.co-cure.org/
Listening to CFIDS – www.wwcoco.com/cfids/
Mary Schweizer's CFIDS pages –
    www.cfids-me.org/marys/essays.html
The CFIDS Association of America – www.cfids.org/
The CFIDS/ME Information Page – www.cfids-me.org/
The CFS Society for Neuroimmunomodulation Research –
    www.square-sun.co.uk/cfs-nim/
The Chronic Syndrome Support Association, Inc. –
    www.cssa-inc.org/index.htm
The National CFIDS Foundation – www.ncf-net.org/

Canada

Nightingale Research Foundation – www.nightingale.ca/

Australia and New Zealand

ANZMES – www.anzmes.org/
Canberra FM-CFS pages –
    www.masmith.inspired.net.au/aus_info/gdlines.htm

ME/Chronic Fatigue Syndrome Society of NSW Inc. – www.zip.com.au/~mesoc/

ME/CFS Australian Support Groups – www.span.com.au/me/

ME-CFS Society (SA) Inc (Australia) – www.sacfs.asn.au/

The Alison Hunter Memorial Foundation – www.ahmf.org/

The ME/Chronic Fatigue Syndrome Society of Victoria Inc. – home.vicnet.net.au/~mecfs/

The ME/CFS Society of Queensland – www.mecfsqld.org.au/

Make
www.thorsonselement.com
your online sanctuary

www.thorsonselement.com

Get online information, inspiration and
guidance to help you on the path to physical
and spiritual well-being. Drawing on the integrity
and vision of our authors and titles, and with
health advice, articles, astrology, tarot, a
meditation zone, author interviews and events
listings, www.thorsonselement.com is a great
alternative to help create space and peace
in our lives.

So if you've always wondered about practising
yoga, following an allergy-free diet, using the
tarot or getting a life coach, we can point you
in the right direction.

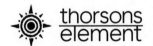

thorsons
element